THERAPEUTIC COMMUNITIES
FOR ADDICTIONS

THERAPEUTIC COMMUNITIES FOR ADDICTIONS

Readings in Theory, Research and Practice

Edited by

GEORGE De LEON, Ph.D.

Phoenix House Foundation
New York, New York

and

JAMES T. ZIEGENFUSS, Jr., Ph.D.

Graduate Program in Public Administration
The Pennsylvania State University
The Capitol Campus
Middletown, Pennsylvania

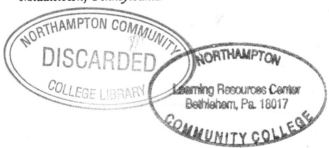
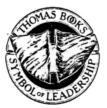

CHARLES C THOMAS • PUBLISHER
Springfield • Illinois • U.S.A.

Published and Distributed Throughout the World by
CHARLES C THOMAS • PUBLISHER
2600 South First Street
Springfield, Illinois 62717

© *1986 by* CHARLES C THOMAS • PUBLISHER
ISBN 0-398-05206-9
Library of Congress Catalog Card Number: 85-24689

Printed in the United States of America
Q-R-3

Library of Congress Cataloging in Publication Data
Main entry under title:

Therapeutic communities for addictions.

Bibliography: p.
1. Substance abuse--Treatment. 2. Therapeutic
community. I. De Leon, George. II. Ziegenfus,
James T. [DNLM: 1. Substance Dependence--rehabilitation.
2. Therapeutic Community. WM 270 T3976]
RC564.T53   1986   616.86   85-24689
ISBN 0-398-05206-9

CONTRIBUTORS

HARRIET BARR, PH.D.

Director of Research

Eagleville Hospital & Rehabilitation Center
Eagleville, Pennsylvania, U.S.A.

D. VINCENT BIASE, PH.D.

Director of Research
Daytop Village
New York, New York, U.S.A.

THOMAS E. BRATTER, ED.D.

President
The John Dewey Academy
Great Barrington, Massachusetts, U.S.A.

EDWARD P. BRATTER

Vice President
The John Dewey Academy
Great Barrington, Massachusetts, U.S.A.

JEROME F.X. CARROLL, PH.D

Director
Partial Hospitalization (Candidate Program)
Eagleville Hospital & Rehabilitation Center
Eagleville, Pennsylvania, U.S.A.

WARD S. CONDELLI, PH.D.

Mid Hudson Psychiatric Center
New Hampton, New York, U.S.A.

GEORGE DE LEON, PH.D.

Director of Research & Evaluation
Phoenix House Foundation
New York, New York, U.S.A.

J. DAVID HAWKINS, PH.D.

Professor & Director, Center for Social Welfare Research
School of Social Work
University of Washington
Seattle, Washington, U.S.A

JESSICA F. HEIMBERG, B.S.

State University at Stony Brook
Stony Brook, New York, U.S.A.

ROBERT D. HINSHELWOOD, M.B. B.S., D.P.M.

Consultant Psychotherapist
St. Bernard's Hospital
Southall, Middlesex, England

SHERRY HOLLAND, M.S.

Director of Research
Gateway Foundation
Chicago, Illinois, U.S.A.

MAXWELL JONES, M.D.

Social Ecologist & Psychiatrist
Nova Scotia, Canada

DAVID H. KERR, M.A.

President
Integrity Inc.
Newark, New Jersey, U.S.A.

MARTIEN KOOYMAN, M.D.

Director
Jellinek Centrum
Amsterdam, Holland

PETER MEYER-FEHR, M.D.

Psychiatric University Hospital
Zurich, Switzerland

D. DWAYNE SIMPSON, PH.D

Professor & Director, Behavioral Research Program
Department of Psychology
Texas A & M University
College Station, Texas, U.S.A.

BERNARD S. SOBEL, D.O.

Director of Psychiatry
Valley Forge Medical Center
Valley Forge, Pennsylvania, U.S.A

BARRY SUGARMAN, PH.D

Lesley College
Cambridge, Massachusetts, U.S.A.

ARTHUR P. SULLIVAN, PH.D

Fordham University
Bronx, New York, U.S.A

NORMAN WACKER, M.A.

Doctoral Candidate
University of Washington
Seattle, Washington, U.S.A

HARRY K. WEXLER, PH.D

New York State Division of Substance Abuse Services
Bureau of Cost Effectiveness & Research
New York, New York, U.S.A.

BARBARA WHEELER, PH.D.

Montclair State College
Montclair, New Jersey, U.S.A.

JAMES T. ZIEGENFUSS, JR., PH.D

Graduate Program in Public Administration
Pennsylvania State University
Middletown, Pennsylvania, U.S.A

DAGMAR ZIMMER-HOEFLER, PH.D.

Social Psychiatric University Hospital
Zurich, Switzerland

PREFACE

THERAPEUTIC communities are well established in addiction and psychiatric services. The concept is international in use, reflecting an ability to cross cultural boundaries. Appropriately, this collection represents current international thinking about the therapeutic community and the addiction problem.

The term therapeutic community connotes a concept, model and methods that are explicitly designed. However, therapeutic communities are social systems, continually adapting and developing. The premise here is that this volume will both document and contribute to that developmental process.

Therapeutic communities have made their most significant contributions to the treatment of addictions. A growing literature records the evolution of the model and, in particular, the advances in research and evaluation. Nevertheless, many workers, professional, lay and academic, remain uninformed as to the nature and impact of therapeutic communities.

The present volume represents a first in a collection of readings on therapeutic communities for substance abuse. Its purpose is to inform audiences from within and outside of the field of addictions of the relevance of this approach in rehabilitating human lives; to strengthen the credibility and efficacy of the therapeutic community within the spectrum of human services, and to further stimulate clinicians, researchers and students to address issues of theory and practice.

The collection itself is representative of the written work on TCs for substance abuse. There were, however, several criteria that entered into the selection of the papers. With few exceptions, all are original manuscripts, written specifically for this volume. Selection attempted to balance research, concepts and issues and include papers from North America and Europe. These focus upon the TC for substance abuse, although several authors are identified with TCs in psychiatric settings because of their implication for addictions work.

ix

The organization of the papers reflects the actual diversity of efforts in the field and development of the therapeutic community approach. The initial set of papers are descriptive of the two main varieties of therapeutic communities, the self-help hierarchical model widely applied to rehabilitating substance abusers, and the so-called democratic model, more commonly implemented for psychiatric patients as well as drug users. Although of somewhat different origins, a rapprochement between these two models is increasingly evident. Section Two contains key papers that document the effectiveness of therapeutic communities in terms of long-term outcomes, and several empirical studies in the important but still underinvestigated area of treatment process. The papers in the last section address emerging issues concerning the future status of the therapeutic community as an established institution within the spectrum of human services. Finally, the Bibliography, though not an exhaustive list of TC studies, contains all references cited in the text and includes selected others.

It is our hope that this volume will demonstrate the broad acceptance of the TC concept and its potential for increased diffusion in the future. There is much work to be done — these papers and the Bibliography of work in the field are but the base for continued efforts.

George De Leon and James Ziegenfuss

CONTENTS

Page

Contributors v

Preface ix
  George De Leon, James T. Ziegenfuss, Jr.

PART I
THE THERAPEUTIC COMMUNITY AS CONCEPT AND MODEL

Chapter

  1. The Therapeutic Community for Substance Abuse: Perspective and
     Approach
       by *George De Leon* 5
  2. Democratic Therapeutic Communities (D.T.C.s) or Programmatic
     Therapeutic Communities (P.T.C.s) or Both?
       by *Maxwell Jones* 19
  3. The Psychodynamics of Therapeutic Communities for Treatment of
     Heroin Addicts
       by *Martien Kooyman* 29
  4. Britain and the Psychoanalytic Tradition in Therapeutic Communities
       by *Robert D. Hinshelwood* 43
  5. The Therapeutic Community: A Codified Concept for Training and
     Upgrading Staff Members Working in a Residential Setting
       by *David H. Kerr* 55
  6. Structure, Variations, and Context: A Sociological View of the
     Therapeutic Community
       by *Barry Sugarman* 65

PART II
RESEARCH AND EVALUATION: OUTCOMES AND PROCESS

  7. Therapeutic Community Research: Overview and Implications
       by *George De Leon* 85

8. Outcome of Drug Abuse Treatment in Two Modalities
    by *Harriet Barr*.. 97
9. 12-Year Follow-up: Outcomes of Opioid Addicts Treated in
   Therapeutic Communities
    by *D. Dwayne Simpson*..109
10. Daytop Miniversity — Phase 2 — College Training in a Therapeutic
    Community — Development of Self Concept Among Drug Free
    Addict/Abusers
    by *D. Vincent Biase, Arthur P. Sullivan and Barbara Wheeler* 121
11. Client Evaluations of Therapeutic Communities and Retention
    by *Ward S. Condelli* 131
12. Side Bets and Secondary Adjustments in Therapeutic Communities
    by *J. David Hawkins & Norman Wacker* 141
13. Motivational Aspects of Heroin Addicts in Therapeutic Communities
    Compared With Those in Other Institutions
    by *Dagmar Zimmer-Hofler & Peter Meyer-Fehr* 157
14. Measuring Process in Drug Abuse Treatment Research
    by *Sherry Holland*...169

PART III
THE FUTURE: ISSUES AND APPLICATION

15. The Therapeutic Community: Looking Ahead
    by *George De Leon* 185
16. Uses and Abuses of Power and Authority Within the American Self-
    Help Residential Therapeutic Community: A Perversion or a Necessity?
    by *Thomas E. Bratter, Edward P. Bratter, & Jessica F. Heimberg*...........191
17. Intergrating Mental Health Personnel and Practices into a
    Therapeutic Community
    by *Jerome F.X. Carroll & Bernard S. Sobel* 209
18. Therapeutic Communities Within Prisons
    by Harry K. Wexler 227
19. Therapeutic Community: A Plan for Continued International
    Development
    by *James T. Ziegenfuss, Jr.* 239

Bibliography 249

THERAPEUTIC COMMUNITIES
FOR ADDICTIONS

Part I

THE THERAPEUTIC COMMUNITY
AS CONCEPT AND MODEL

CHAPTER 1

THE THERAPEUTIC COMMUNITY FOR SUBSTANCE ABUSE: PERSPECTIVE AND APPROACH

GEORGE DE LEON

SINCE THE 1960s, the spectrum of drug abusers has widened. Differences among users in drug abuse patterns, lifestyle, and motivation for change are addressed by four major treatment modalities — detoxification, methadone maintenance, drug free outpatient and drug free residential therapeutic communities (TCs). Each modality has its view of substance abuse and each impacts the drug abuser in different ways.

The TC views drug abuse as a deviant behavior, reflecting impeded personality development and/or chronic deficits in social, educational and economic skills. Its antecedents lie in socio-economic disadvantage, poor family effectiveness and in psychological factors. Thus, the principal aim of the therapeutic community is a global change in lifestyle; abstinence from illicit substances, elimination of antisocial activity, employability, pro-social attitudes and values. The rehabilitative approach requires multi-dimensional influence and training which for most can only occur in a 24-hour residental setting.

The therapeutic community can be distinguished from other major drug treatment modalities in two fundamental ways. *First*, the primary "therapist" and teacher in the TC is the community itself consisting of peers and staff who, as role models of successful personal change, serve as guides in the recovery process. Thus, the community provides a 24-hour learning experience in which individual changes in conduct, attitudes and emotions are monitored and mutually reinforced in the daily regime.

Second, unlike other modalities, TCs offer a systematic approach to achieve its main rehabilitative objective, which is guided by an explicit perspective on the drug abuse disorder, the client, and recovery.

This paper outlines the therapeutic community approach to rehabilitation. The initial section provides an overview of the TC, its background and perspective on rehabilitation. The second section draws a picture of the TC approach in terms of its basic elements and the stages of treatment.

OVERVIEW

Background: Therapeutic communities for substance abuse appeared a decade later than did therapeutic communities in psychiatric settings pioneered by Jones and others in the United Kingdom.

The two models evolved in parallel independence reflecting differences in their philosophy, social organization, clients served and therapeutic processes. Jones explains that the therapeutic community referred to a movement which originated in psychiatry in the United Kingdom at the end of World War II. It was "an attempt to establish a democratic system in hospitals where the domination of the doctors in a traditional hierarchy system was replaced by open communication, information sharing, decision making by consensus and problem solving sharing, as far as possible, with all patients and staff," (Jones, 1953). The name therapeutic community evolved in these settings.

The therapeutic community for substance abuse emerged in the 1960s as a self-help alternative to existing conventional treatments. Unhelped by the medical and correctional establishments, recovering alcoholics and drug addicts were its first participant-developers. Though its modern antecedents can be traced to Alcoholics Anonymous and Synanon, the TC prototype is ancient, existing in all forms of communal healing and support. Today, the term "therapeutic community" is generic, describing a variety of drug free residential programs. About a quarter of these conform to the traditional long term model. These have made the greatest impact upon rehabilitating substance abusers.

The Traditional TC: Traditional therapeutic communities are similar in planned duration of stay (15-24 months), structure, staffing pattern, perspective and in rehabilitative regime, although they differ in size (30-600 beds) and client demographies. Staff are a mixture of TC trained clinicians and human service professionals. Primary clinical staff are usually former substance abusers who themselves were rehabilitated in TC programs. Ancillary staff consist of professionals in mental health vocational, educational, family counseling, fiscal, administration and legal services.

TCs accommodate a broad spectrum of drug abusers. Although it originally attracted narcotic addicts, a majority of their client populations are non-opioid abusers. Thus, this modality has responded to the changing trend in drug use patterns, treating clients with drug problems of varying severity, different lifestyles, and various social, economic and ethnic backgrounds.

Clients in traditional programs are usually male (75%) and in their mid-twenties (50%). TCs are almost all racially mixed, and most are age-integrated, with 25 percent of their clients under 21, although a few TCs have separate facilities for adolescents. About half of all admissions are from broken homes or ineffective families, and more than three quarters have been arrested at some time in their lives.

The TC Perspective: Full accounts of the TC perspective are described elsewhere (Deitch & Zweben, 1976, 1979; De Leon, 1981, 1984a, 1985; De Leon & Beschner, 1977; De Leon & Rosenthal, 1979; Kaufman & De Leon, 1978). Although expressed in a social psychological idiom, this perspective evolved directly from the experience of recovering participants in therapeutic communities.

Drug abuse is viewed as a disorder of the whole person, affecting some or all areas of functioning. Cognitive and behavioral problems appear, as do mood disturbances. Thinking may be unrealistic or disorganized; values are confused, nonexistent or antisocial. Frequently there are deficits in verbal, reading, writing and marketable skills. And, whether couched in existential or psychological terms, moral or even spiritual issues are apparent.

Abuse of any substance is viewed as over-determined behavior. Physiological dependency is secondary to the wide range of influences which control the individual's drug use behavior. Invariably, problems and situations associated with discomfort become regular signals for resorting to drug use. For some abusers, physiological factors may be important but for most these remain minor relative to the functional deficits which accumulate with continued substance abuse. Physical addiction or dependency must be seen in the wider context of the individual's life.

Thus, the problem is the person, not the drug. Addiction is a symptom, not the essense of the disorder. In the TC, chemical detoxification is a condition of entry, not a goal of treatment. Rehabilitation focuses upon maintaining a drug free existence.

Rather than drug use patterns, individuals are distinguished along dimensions of psychological dysfunction and social deficits. Many clients have never acquired conventional lifestyles. Vocational and educational problems are marked; middle class mainstream values are either missing or unachievable. Usually these clients emerge from a socially disadvantaged sector, where drug abuse is more a social response than a psychological disturbance. Their TC experience is better termed habilitation, the development of a socially productive, conventional lifestyle for the first time in their lives.

Among clients from more advantaged backgrounds, drug abuse is more directly expressive of psychological disorder or existential malaise, and the word rehabilitation is more suitable, emphasizing a return to a lifestyle previously lived, known, and perhaps rejected.

Nevertheless, substance abusers in TCs share important similarities. Either as cause or consequence of their drug abuse, all reveal features of personality disturbance and/or impeded social function. Thus, all residents in the TC follow the same regime. Individual differences are recognized in specific treatment plans that modify the emphasis, not the course, of their experience in the therapeutic community.

In the TC's view of recovery, the aim of rehabilitation is global. The primary psychological goal is to change the negative patterns of behavior, thinking and feeling that predispose drug use; the main social goal is to develop a responsible drug free lifestyle. Stable recovery, however, depends upon a successful integration of these social and psychological goals. For example, healthy behavioral alternatives to drug use are reinforced by commitment to the values of abstinence; acquiring vocational or educational skills and social productivity is motivated by the values of achievement and self-reliance. Behavioral change is unstable without insight, and insight is insufficient without felt experience. Thus, conduct, emotions, skills, attitudes and values must be integrated to insure enduring change.

The rehabilitative regime is shaped by several broad assumptions about recovery.

Motivation: Recovery depends upon positive and negative pressures to change. Some clients seek help, driven by stressful external pressures, others are moved by more intrinsic factors. For all, however, remaining in treatment requires continued motivation to change. Thus, elements of the rehabilitation approach are designed to sustain motivation, or detect early signs of premature termination.

Self Help: Although the influence of treatment depends upon the person's motivation and readiness, change does not occur in a vacuum. The individual must permit the impact of treatment or learning to occur. Thus, rehabilitation unfolds as an interaction between the client and the therapeutic environment.

Social Learning: A lifestyle change occurs in a social context. Negative patterns, attitudes and roles were not acquired in isolation, nor can they be altered in isolation. Thus, recovery depends not only upon what has been learned, but how and where learning occurs. This assumption is the basis for the community itself serving as teacher. Learning is active, by doing and participating. A socially responsible role is acquired by acting the role. What is learned is identified with the people involved in the learning process, with peer support and staff, as credible role models. Because newly acquired ways of coping are threatened by isolation and its potential for relapse. A perspective on self, society and life must be affirmed by a network of others.

Treatment as an Episode: Residency is a relatively brief period in an individual's life, and its influence must compete with the influence of the years before and after treatment. For this reason, unhealthy "outside" influences are minimized until the individuals are better prepared to engage these on their own and the treatment regime is designed for high impact. Thus, life in the TC is necessarily intense, its daily regime demanding, its therapeutic confrontations unmoderated.

THE TC APPROACH

A. TC Structure

TCs are stratified communities composed of peer groups that hold memberships in wider aggregates that are led by individual staff. Together they constitute the community, or family, in a residential facility. This peer-to-community structure strengthens the individual's identification with a perceived, ordered network of others. More importantly, it arranges relationships of mutual responsibility to others at various levels of the program.

The operation of the community itself is the task of the residents, working under staff supervision. Work assignments, called job functions, are arranged in a hierarchy, according to seniority, individual progress and productivity. The new client enters a setting of upward mobility. Job assignments begin with the most menial tasks (e.g., mopping the floor) and lead vertically to levels of coordination and management. Indeed, clients come in as patients and can leave as staff. This social organization reflects the fundamental aspects of the rehabilitative approach, mutual self help, work as therapy, peers as role models and staff as rational authorities.

Mutual Self Help: The essential dynamic in the TC is mutual self help. Thus, the day to day activities of a therapeutic community are conducted by the residents themselves. In their jobs, groups, meetings, recreation, personal and social time, it is residents who continually transmit to each other the main messages and expectations of the community.

The extent of the self help process in the TC is evident in the broad range of resident job assignments. These include conducting all house services (e.g., cooking, cleaning, kitchen service, minor repair), serving as apprentices and running all departments, conducting meetings and peer encounter groups.

The TC is managed as an autocracy, with staff serving as rational authorities. Their psychological relationship with the residents is as role models and parental surrogates, who foster the self help, developmental process through managerial and clinical means. They monitor and evaluate client status, supervise resident groups, assign and supervise resident job functions and oversee house operations. Clinically, staff conduct all therapeutic groups, provide individual counseling, organize social and recreational projects and confer with significant others. They decide matters of resident status, discipline, promotion, transfers, discharges, furloughs, and treatment planning.

Work as Education and Therapy: In the TC, work mediates essentail educational and therapeutic effects. Vertical job movements carry the obvious rewards of status and privilege. However, lateral job changes are more frequent, providing exposure to all aspects of the community. Typically, residents experience many lateral job changes that enable them to learn new skills and to negotiate the system. This increased involvement also heightens their sense of belonging and affirms their commitment to the community.

Job changes in the TC are singularly effective therapeutic tools, providing both measures of, and incentives for, behavioral and attitudinal change. In the vertical structure of the TC, ascendency marks how well the client has assimilated what the community teaches and expects, hence, the job promotion is an explicit measure of the resident's improvement and growth.

Conversely, lateral or downward job movements also create situations that require demonstrations of personal growth. A resident may be removed from one job to a lateral position in another department or dropped back to a lower status position for clinical reasons. These movements are designed to teach new ways of coping with reversals and change that appear to be unfair or arbitrary.

Peers as Role Models: People are the essential ingredient in the therapeutic community. Peers as role models and staff as role models and rational authorities are the primary mediators of the recovery process.

Indeed, the strength of the community as a context for social learning relates to the number and quality of its role models. All members of the community are expected to be role models — roommates, older and younger residents, junior, senior and directorial staff. TCs require these multiple role models to maintain the integrity of the community and assure the spread of social learning effects.

Residents who demonstrate the expected behaviors and reflect the values and teachings of the community are viewed as role models. This is illustrated in two main attributes.

Role models "act as if." They behave as the person they should be, rather than as the person they have been. Despite resistance, perceptions or feelings to the contrary, they engage in the expected behavior and consistently maintain the attitudes and values of the community. These include self motivation, commitment to work and striving, positive regard for staff as authority and an optimistic outlook toward the future.

In the TC's view, "acting as if" has significance beyond conformity. It is an essential mechanism for more complete psychological change. Feelings, insights and altered self-perceptions often **follow** rather than precede behavior change.

Role models display responsible concern. This concept is closely akin to the notion of, "I am my brother's keeper." Showing responsible concern involves willingness to confront others whose behavior is not in keeping with the rules of the TC, the spirit of the community or the knowledge which is consistent with growth and rehabilitation. Role models are obligated to be aware of the appearance, attitude, moods and performances of their peers, and confront negative signs in these. In particular, role models are aware of their own behavior in overall community and the process prescribed for personal growth.

Staff as Rational Authorities: TC clients often have had difficulties with authorities, who have not been trusted or perceived as guides and teachers. Thus, they need a successful experience with a rational authority who is credible (recovered), supportive, correcting and protecting, in order to gain authority over themselves (personal autonomy). Implicit in their role as rational authorities, staff provide the reasons for their decisions and the meaning of consequences. They exercise their powers to train and guide, facilitate and correct, rather than punish, control or exploit.

B. Daily Regime: Basic Elements

The daily regime is full and varied. Although designed to facilitate the management of the community, its scope and schedule reflect an understanding of the conditions of drug abuse. It provides an orderly environment for many who customarily have lived in chaotic or disruptive settings; it reduces boredom and distracts from negative preoccupations which have, in the past, been associated with drug use; and it offers opportunity to achieve satisfaction from a busy schedule and the completion of daily chores.

The typical day in a therapeutic community is highly structured, beginning with a 7 PM wakeup and ending at 11 PM in the evening. It includes a variety of meetings, job functions (work therapy), therapeutic groups, recreation and individual counseling. These activities contribute to the TC process and may be grouped into three main elements, community enhancement, therapeutic-educative, community and clinical management.

Community Enhancement Element: These activities, which facilitate assimilation into the community, include the four main facility-wide meetings: the morning meeting, seminar and house meeting, held each day, and the general meeting, which is called when needed.

Morning meeting: All residents of the facility and the staff on premises assemble after breakfast, usually for 30 to 45 minutes. The purpose is to initiate the daily activities with a positive attitude, motivate residents and strengthen unity. This meeting is particularly important in that most residents of TCs have never adapted to the routine of an ordinary day.

Seminars convene every afternoon, usually for 1 to 1½ hours. The seminar collects all the residents together at least once during the working day. Thus, staff observation of the entire facility is regularized since the seminar in the afternoon complements the daily morning meetings, and the house meeting in the evening. A clinical aim of the seminar, however, is to balance the individual's emotional and cognitive experience. Of the various meetings and group processes in the TC, the seminar is unique in its emphasis upon listening, speaking and conceptual behavior.

House meetings convene nightly, after dinner, usually for one hour. The main aim of these meetings is to transact community business, although they also have a clinical objective. In this forum, social pressure is judiciously employed to facilitate individual change through public acknowledgement of positive or negative behaviors among certain individuals or subgroups.

General meetings convene only when needed to address negative behavior, attitudes or incidents in the facility. All residents and staff (including those not on duty) are assembled at any time and for indefinite duration. These meetings, conducted by staff, are designed to identify problem people or conditions, to reaffirm motivation and reinforce positive behavior and attitudes. A variety of techniques may be employed, e.g., special sessions to relieve guilt, staff lecturing and testimony, dispensing sanctions for individuals or groups.

Therapeutic-Educative Element: These activities consist of various groups and staff counseling. This element focuses on individual issues. It provides an exclusive setting for expressing feelings for resolution of personal and business issues in the evening. It trains communication and interpersonal relating skills; examines and confronts the behaviors and attitudes displayed in the various roles of the clients; offers instruction in alternate modes of behavior.

There are four main forms of group activity in the TC: encounters, probes, marathons and tutorials. These differ somewhat in format, aims and methods, but all attempt to foster trust and peer solidarity in order to facilitate personal disclosure, insight and therapeutic change.

Peer encounter is the cornerstone of group process in the TC. The term "encounter" is generic, describing a variety of forms which utilize confrontational procedures as their main approach. Encounter groups meet at least three times weekly, usually in the evening, for two hours. Although its process is intense, its aim is modest, to heighten the individual's awareness of the images, attitudes and conduct that should be modified.

Probes meet as needed, usually in the early months of residency. These groups, which last 4 to 8 hours, aim to strengthen trust and identification with others; and to increase the staff's understanding of important background of the person.

Marathons are extended group sessions that meet as needed, usually for 24 to 30 hours, to initiate a process of resolution of life experiences that have impeded the individual's growth or development. Marathons make liberal use of dramatic, visual, auditory and environmental props to facilitate a "working through" of deeper emotional experiences.

Tutorial groups meet regularly and are primarily directed toward training or teaching. Three major themes of tutorials are personal growth concepts, (e.g., self reliance, independence, relationships); job skill training, (e.g., managing a department or the reception desk); clinical skills training (e.g., use of the encounter tools).

The important differences across these groups are in leadership, objectives, material used and approach. All but the encounter groups are led by staff, with the help of senior residents.

The focus of the encounter is behavioral, its approach is confrontational; its material draws upon peer and staff observation of the individual's daily conduct. Probes go much beyond the here and now behavioral incident, which is the primary material of the encounter, to the events and experiences of the individual's history. Although certain encounter tools are utilized, (e.g., identification, prodding), the main techniques of the probe are conversational but may include role playing or other methods to reduce defensiveness and resistance to strong emotional memories. Rather than confrontation, the probe emphasizes the use of support, understanding and empathy. The main distinctions between the probe and the marathon are length, intensity of therapeutic intervention and goals. The probe may be employed as a regular clinical intervention or to prepare the individual for the marathon. Another difference lies in the range of techniques and paraphernalia which are used. Tutorials emphasize teaching, which contrasts with the confrontation of the encounter to correct behavior or the methods in probes and marathons to facilitate emotional catharsis and insight.

The four basic groups are supplemented by others that convene as needed. These vary in focus, format and composition. For example, gender, ethnic or age-specific groups may utilize encounter, tutorial or probe formats; dormitory, room or departmental encounters will address issues of daily community living.

Counseling: One-to-one counseling further balances the needs of the individual with those of the community. Peer exchange is ongoing, frequent and constitutes the most consistent counseling in TCs. However, staff counseling sessions are conducted on an as needed basis, usually informally. The staff counseling method in the TC is not traditional, evident in its main features: interpersonal sharing, direct support, minimal interpretation, didactic instruction and encounter.

Community-Clinical Management Element: The objective of these activities is to protect the community as a whole and to strengthen it as a context for social learning. The main activities consist of privileges and disciplinary sanctions.

Privilege: In the TC, privileges are explicit rewards that reinforce the value of earned achievement. Privileges are accorded by behavior, attitude change, job performance and overall clinical progress in the program. Displays of inappropriate behavior or negative attitude can result in loss of some or all privileges, offering the resident the opportunity to earn them back by showing improvement.

Privileges acquire their importance because they are **earned**. The earning process requires investment of time, energy, self modification, risk of failure and disappointment. Thus, the earning process establishes the value of privileges and hence their potency as social reinforcements.

The type of privilege is related to clinical progress and time in program, ranging from phone and letter writing in early treatment to overnight furloughs in later treatment. Successful movement through each stage earns privileges that grant wider personal lattitude and increased self responsibility.

Discipline and Sanctions: Therapeutic communities have their own specific rules and regulations that guide the behavior of residents and the management of facilities. Their explicit purpose is to ensure the safety and health of the community; their implicit aim is to train and teach residents through the use of discipline.

In the TC, social and physical safety are prerequisites for psychological trust. Thus, sanctions are invoked against any behavior which threatens the safety of the therapeutic environment. For example, breaking the TC's cardinal rules — no violence or the threat of violence, verbal or gestural — can bring immediate expulsion. Even minor house rules are addressed, such as stealing mundane sundries (toothbrushes, books, etc.).

The choice of sanction depends upon the severity of the infraction, time in program and history of infractions. For example, verbal reprimands, loss of privileges, speaking bans, may be selected for less severe infractions; job demotions, loss of residential time or expulsion may be invoked for more serious infractions. These measures (contracts) vary in duration from 3 to perhaps 21 days and are re-evaluated by staff and peers in terms of their efficacy.

Though often perceived as punitive, the basic purpose of contracts is to provide a learning experience through compelling residents to attend to their own conduct, to reflect on their own motivation, to feel some consequence of their behavior and to consider alternate forms of acting under stimilar situations.

Contracts also have important community functions. The entire facility is made aware of disciplinary actions that have been taken with any resident. Thus, contracts act as deterrents against violations; they provide vicarious learning experiences in others; and as symbols of safety and integrity, they strengthen community cohesiveness.

C. The TC Process

Rehabilation in the TC unfolds as a developmental process occurring in a social learning context. Values, conducts, emotions and cognitive understanding (insight) must be integrated in the evolution of a socially responsible, personally autonomous individual.

The developmental process itself can be understood as a passage through three main stages of incremental learning; the learning which occurs at each stage facilitates change at the next and each change reflects increased maturity and personal autonomy.

Stage I (Induction — 0 to 60 days): The main goal of this initial phase of residency are assessment of individual needs and orientation to the TC. Important differences among clients generally do not appear until they experience some reduction in the circumstantial stress usually present at entry and have had some interaction with the treatment regime. Thus, observation of the individual continues during the initial residential period to identify special problems in their adaptation to the TC.

The goal of orientation in the initial phase of residency is to assimilate the individual into the community through full participation and involvement in all of its activities. Rapid assimilation is crucial at this point, when clients are most ambivalent about the long tenure of residency. Thus, the new resident is immediately involved in the daily residential regime. Emphasis, however, is placed not upon treatment but upon education and role induction into the community process. Therapeutic and educational activities focus on the TC perspective, its approach and the rationale for long term residential treatment.

Stage II (Primary Treatment — 2 to 12 Months): During this state, main TC objectives of socialization, personal growth and psychological awareness are pursued through all of the therapeutic and community activities. Primary treatment actually consists of three phases separated by natural landmarks in the socialization-developmental process. Phases roughly correlate with time in program (1 to 4 months, 5 to 8 months and 9 to 12 months). These periods are marked by plateaus of stable behavior which signal futher change.

In each phase the daily regime of meetings, work, recreation and therapeutic groups remains the same. However, progress is reflected in the client's profile at the end of each phase, which can be typified in terms of three interrelated dimensions, community status, developmental and psychological change. Community status describes the degree to which residents have acquired the attributes of the role model, measured mainly in their job functions and privileges. The developmental dimension describes the degree to which residents have altered their drug involved profile, in conduct, language, attitude and outlook. This is mainly reflected in the extent to which they have internalized the TC's perspective and commitment to change. The psychological dimension describes the degree to which residents reveal personal growth, e.g., maturity, openness, insight-self awareness; emotional stability and self esteem.

Stage III (Re-Entry — 13 to 24 Months): Re-entry is the stage at which the client must strengthen skills for autonomous decision-making and the capacity for self-management with less reliance on rational authorities or a well-formed peer network. There are two phases of the re-entry stage.

Early Re-Entry (13 to 18 Months): The main goal of this phase, during which clients continue to live in the facility, is preparation for healthy separation from the community.

Emphasis upon rational authority decreases under the assumption that the client has acquired a sufficient degree of self-management. This is reflected in more individual decision-making about privileges, social plans and life design. The group process involves fewer leaders at this stage, fewer encounters and more shared decision-making. Particular emphasis is placed upon life skills seminars, which provide didactic training for life outside the community. Attendance is mandated for sessions on budgeting, job seeking, use of alcohol, sexuality, parenting, use of leisure time, etc.

During this stage, individal plans are a collective task of the client, a key staff member and peers. These plans are actually blue-prints of educational and vocational programs, which include goal attainment schedules, methods of improving inter-personal and family relationships, as well as social and sexual behavior. Clients may be attending school or holding full-time jobs either within or outside the TC at this point. Still, they are expected to participate in house activities when possible and carry some community responsibilities (e.g., facility coverage at night).

Late Re-Entry (18 to 24 Months): The goal of this phase is to complete a successful separation from residency. Clients are on "live-out" status, involved in full-time jobs or education, maintaining their own households, usually with live-out peers. They may attend such aftercare services as A.A., N.A. or take part in family or individual therapy. This phase is viewed as the end of residency, but not of program participation. Contact with the program is frequent at first and only gradually reduced to weekly phone calls and monthly visits with a primary counselor.

Completion marks the end of active program involvement. Graduation itself, however, is an annual event conducted in the facility, for completees at least a year beyond their residency.

Thus, the therapeutic community experience is preparation rather than cure. Residence in the program facilitates a process of change that must continue throughout life, and what is learned in treatment are the tools to guide the individual on a steady path of continued change. Completion, or graduation, therefore, is not an end, but a beginning.

CHAPTER 2

DEMOCRATIC THERAPEUTIC COMMUNITIES (D.T.C.s) OR PROGRAMMATIC THERAPEUTIC COMMUNITIES (P.T.C.s) OR BOTH?

MAXWELL JONES

A NTHONY GLASER suggested that the two types of Therapeutic Community (T.C.), which serve different functions, often are confused because both use the same designation TC (Glaser, 1983). He suggests the name Democractic TC (D.T.C.) for the one linked to psychiatry which uses almost exclusively trained professionals from medicine, psychology, social work, etc. And Programmatic TC (P.T.C.) for the units designed for drug and alcohol addiction and which employ mainly ex-addicts as staff. The characteristics of the two TCs have been described many times; DTCs by Jones (1976) and PTC's by De Leon (1974).

Unlike Glaser, I feel that there are some interesting similarities between the two TCs, as well as major differences as follows:

1. Both aim to achieve an integrated "family identity" but with considerable differences in the quality of feelings, as though we were comparing the Church of Rome with say the Quakers: one feels the difference immediately, but it is difficult to describe the subjective feelings involved.

2. Both care about clients and staff. With DTCs this is at a relatively intimate interpersonal level with staff, and rather parental in quality between staff and patients, and more or less spontaneous among the clients (patients). With PTCs there is an awesome intensity, dedication, and militarism throughout the system. No one appears to question the nature or seriousness of the task — to buck the drug addiction which has

pushed all other issues family, friends, work, etc., aside. It was as though the individual housed a virtual stranger inside him, and survival was only possible if the stranger could be eradicated.

I want to review the nature and characteristics of these two largely disparate TCs.

DTCs evolved from a treatment enviroment designed to change antisocial behavior, starting in 1947. My colleagues and I undertook to try and help the "down and outs" in London — a mixed bag of social problems including chronic unemployment, deviancy and antisocial behavior, spilling over into mental illness and crime. This project was housed in an old workhouse on the outskirts of London with accommodation for 100 clients of both sexes. There were social pressures of various kinds — predominantly society's distrust and dislike for "deviants," but also psychiatry's resistance to "psychopathic personality," which resulted in an increasing referral rate of individuals with this label (diagnosis) to fill the new facility. The courts, too, wanted an alternative to a prison sentence.

For this paper, I restrict my study of DTCs to these clients. I ignore the medical use of the term therapeutic community which means any type of psychiatric disorder undergoing treatment, which utilizes large or small group settings in a democratic social organization. This contrasts with the traditional medical hierarchical social system with a formal doctor/patient relationship, and with an emphasis on pharmacotherapy and physical treatment methods.

In this way instead of comparing apples and oranges when talking of DTCs and PTCs, one is essentially looking at two very different approaches to the treatment of personality disorders, which PTCs are recognizing as a treatment challenge in addition to the drug addiction itself. To quote O'Brien and Biase (1981),

> "The theory underlying the traditional therapeutic community approach views drug addiction and abuse as being largely symptomatic psychological character disorder and/or privation alienation. Abuse behavior resulting primarily from the former is assumed to stem from or be exacerbated by faulty sociopsychological development."

This statement could refer equally well to the core clinical material in either DTCs or PTCs and what is meant by "The traditional therapeutic community approach" is unclear. Does it refer to the early work at Henderson Hospital in the 40s or 50s or to the current view held by some PTCs? The state that "such compulsive and destructive behavior is viewed as stunted and immature in the context of psychosocial development." This has been the basis of our theoretical position for at least three decades in attempting to understand the anomaly of emotional growth (as opposed to the growth of intelligence) in character disorders. A character disorder may have an I.Q. (intelligence quotient) at the highest level of testing, but at the same time show an emotional level or social maturity equivalent to that of a 3 year old child (Jones, 1962).

O'Brien and Biase outline the specific methods used to ameliorate this drug abuse and personality disorder beginning with removal from the client's natural environment to a residential setting (a PTC). In this "family setting" away from negative outside influences "Through the forces of group dynamics his/her own behavioral and interpersonal relationships are revealed." Their use of the term group dynamics is based largely on role modelling a set of rules. This philosophy of behavior which each PTC has evolved is thought to be essentially similar in all PTCs. This system of values, attitudes and beliefs reflects a summation of addicts' experience over time in relation to personality defenses against the problem of addiction. It is *their* treatment policy expounded by the staff, mostly ex-addicts, who, themselves, went through a similar experience as residents, and now promulgate an identical philosophy to new residents. This process, although it is central to the whole treatment plan, is difficult to conceptualize. Maybe it amounts to a mix of persuasion, role modelling in response to a need, primary conditioning with strong reinforcement for conformity to unit culture and learning theory? If the latter, it is more related to rote learning or operant conditioning than to the social learning of DTC's where interacting in a group setting raises many divergent views for discussion. The group process or group dynamics is essentially one of incorporation by the individual or individuals of some new but compatible concepts with a resulting attitude change, in the individual or group. I will return to this subject of social learning later when discussing DTC's. This persuasive process in PTCs, as described, is a direct descendent of the Alcoholics Anonymous (AA) regime, and, in fact, Synanon, the first PTC, was started 23 years after AA by Charles E. Dederich, a graduate of AA. While AA is based on a belief system that is essentially religious, PTCs started as a secular system. Glaser (1974) describes the change as one from theology to sociology. Interesting enough, it seems that Synanon now perceives itself as a religion in its own right!

PTC's have a hierarchical social organization which means that the power and authority are in the hands of the leader or leaders. Glaser's article (1974) on the historical development of PTCs points to a long line of authoritative figures. Glaser shows how AA was strongly influenced by the Oxford Group Movement led by a Lutheran minister, Dr. Frank Buckman. There seems to be an astonishing continuity of this evangelism from the intense religiosity of the Middle Ages to the present secular ideologies of which PTC is one example. In a rather similar way psychoanalytic beliefs held by some staff in DTCs may reflect in part archytypical beliefs from antiquity, giving the psychotherapist some of the qualities of a witch doctor. Glaser's research certainly helps to explain some aspects of the belief system of persuasiveness found in PTC's and, in particular, the confrontation used routinely in encounter groups. O'Brien and Biase (1981) recognize the danger of the abuse of authority in a hierarchical system such as a PTC and applaud the introduction of a nationwide Code of Ethnics to safeguard client rights.

Allied to the abuse of authority is the problem of coercion, which on occasion may amount to violence. It is here that PTCs and DTCs differ most markedly and the label "totalitarism" may be directed at PTCs. Deitch and Zweben (1984) have written on this subject, and emphasize the delicate balance implicit in the ideology of a PTC, especially the coercive techniques employed immediately following admission. They point out that at this early stage of induction the ground is set for the later bonding between staff and clients which is central to a successful outcome. But the coercive pressures implicit in encounter-type groups, which emphasize mandatory requirements if residence is to continue, can backfire. The unfamiliar and intimindating experience of staff and peers shouting obscenities, etc., at the client for failure to comply to some mandatory behavior can contribute to "splitting" at an early stage. Other forms of coercion such as bullying and threatening can be used by the group. In fact, De Leon (1983) has shown that at Phoenix House in New York only 23 percent of clients survive the first year and 15 percent complete the course (usually 2 years). Dietch and Zweben conclude that to break down character defenses and enhance impulse control in these addicts with personality disorders, it is essential to use coercive methods — but only within certain limits, or they run the risk of clients "splitting."

Both the abuse of power and the use of coercion may lead to public criticism. Often overlooked are the potentially therapeutic qualities which they may involve — if used appropriately. Glaser (1971) argues convincingly that at Gaudeuzia, a PTC in Philadelphia, extensive use is made of existentialism as a treatment philosophy. A person is what he does — his behavior defines what he is, rather than what is usually assumed, his words, thoughts and feelings. It follows that man has to assume responsibility for his behavior and cannot blame adversity for his drug addiction or other failings. But he also has the capacity to change his behavior for the better, and he has to assume responsibility for this reversal; he cannot fall back on excuses such as "sickness."

PTCs make extensive use of other behavior modification techniques, especially operant conditioning. Here positive (good) behavior is rewarded and negative (bad) behavior is punished. So socially acceptable behavior in a PTC leads to an improved status in the PTC hierarchy; the peak of success is being admitted to the position of staff member. On the other hand, failure to conform to the rules of the PTC leads to public denounciation and loss of status.

Treatment in a DTC follows very different lines compared with a PTC. Instead of existentialism and operant conditioning, there is the use of individual, group or community psychotherapy, and systems theory. There is not the same consistency in the treatment pattern that characterizes the PTCs and this is inevitable in view of the fact the DTCs operate in virtually all types of psychiatric treatment facilities with the whole spectrum of mentally ill patients. I have limited myself to those DTCs that treat personality or character disorders; patients like most personality types in the PTCs. This makes a comparison between the two systems much less complex.

The primary goal in PTCs is to eliminate the drug habit. Even a successful result may not have eliminated the personality disorder leaving a treatment need (O'Brien and Biase, 1981).

The treatment philosophy that my colleagues and I have developed over the years stems from group therapy and systems theory (Jones, 1982). We have used a very simple form of group treatment at a largely conscious level, not delving into childhood experiences, dreams, etc. The term "group therapy" implies a group of people who, in an optimal environment with a leader or leaders skilled in psychodynamics, interact for the purpose of conflict resolution and social maturation. For such a process to occur, regularly scheduled meetings over an extended period of time are essential. This is the stand taken by most group psychotherapists whose basic training included an extensive knowledge of Freudian psychodynamics and/or object relations theory.

As with any relatively new discipline, universal standards of training and practice have not yet been formulated, but there is general agreement that a mix of didactic and experiential experiences is essential. Until we understand the details of group process more fully, it is inevitable that psychoanalytic theory remains the basis of didactic training and secondly, that some form of exposure to actual group process is part of a group therapist's "apprenticeship" (Roman, and Porter, 1978). Intellectual understanding of group phenomena is not enough.

Perhaps the most intriguing part of group therapy is the way it forces one to recognize nuances of interpersonal behavior that are usually missed. It is a depth perspective where the spoken word is no longer the pre-eminent aspect of communication but only a part. There is a subtle process at work in the group where members begin to identify themselves with the group and place increasing trust in it. This build up of trust is partly the result of the group's performance in assuming responsibility for its members and partly due to other more intangible factors of an archetypal kind, e.g., man's need for a family or social support system which is evident throughout history. Little is as yet understood about intuition, but it is linked with philosophy and religion from many cultures. Further research in this area is needed. At a more tangible level we know that the wisdom of the group can amount to more than the total inputs of the individuals concerned — this synergism links group therapy with education and growth. I have avoided a detailed discussion of therapy as this is available in the many publications in this field (Yalom, 1975).

As with PTCs large daily groups lasting about an hour are the rule. These entail frequent, preferably daily, meetings of all patients and staff where the patients experience a supportive environment, which encourages communication of both content and feeling. The role of the staff is to open the door for such information sharing, by their relationship skills, both natural and acquired through training. If these are largely absent, the patient/staff meeting (or community meeting as it is often called) will come to be dreaded by both patients and staff because "nothing happens" and no one's self image is enhanced. In brief, no group is better than the people in it. But if the relationship skills of the staff have already been assured by appropriate selection of individuals who can stand the scrutiny of their performance in these daily community meetings, and have a basic training in group dynamics, systems theory, and psychotherapy, then something positive does begin to emerge.

The process of change in the direction of a more effective use of the social environment (the community meeting representing a microcosm of the ward life) is greatly helped by a daily staff process review of the community meeting, immediately following the patient-staff meeting. In my experience, staff usually try to avoid what is potentially a painful learning situation. The doctor may be too busy, or the nurses express a concern to get back to the patients (by having coffee in the nursing station well insulated from the patients!).

My preference is to attempt to "process" the meeting. How did it start? Did patients and staff arrive in time? Who spoke first? etc. All staff have been exposed to the same interactional situation but will react individually according to their personalities, training, and status. In order to catch the process of change, the sequence of events, e.g., content at both conceptual and feeling levels, non-verbal communication, the emotional climate of the meeting, themes which "catch on" and involve everyone, nonsequitors, avoidance mechansims by both patients and staff, have all to be relived as far as possible.

Resistance to such a detailed scrutiny of staff performance can take subtle forms — an amusing anecdote about a patient which is not related to the "here and now" of the meeting, deferential respect for the status of staff members which inhibits the free flow of communication, the silence expected of the new staff member especially in the lower status levels, fear of not saying the "right thing" or of ridicule, are all common. After all, who wants to have his or her performance scrutinized daily? It is only people who are motivated to learn, and welcome an opportunity to see themselves through other people's eyes. We are approaching the concept of a therapeutic culture where criticism is linked with a positive function of growth and not the negative "put down" function commonly attributed to this term.

In brief, I have tried to touch on the dynamics of change and learning which can emerge from a daily scrutiny of staff/patient interaction in a community meeting followed by a staff review, preferably lasting as long as the community meeting. To me this represents a training opportunity par excellence, often avoided because learning is a painful process.

Clearly the success of such reviews is dependent on many variables not elaborated here. The quality of training of the staff, the nature of the patient population, the sanctions of the governing body, and above all the skill, enthusiasm and integrity of the leader or leaders, is of paramount importance.

Given a social organization based on interaction at ward level, many other aspects of a flexible social system follow. Staff meetings to examine the attitudes, feelings and beliefs of the various staff members will usually lead to an examination of the authority structure, delegation of responsibility, and authority to the system (including the patients), shared decision-making, consensus, and so on. The model that emerges will inevitably reflect the attitudes of the staff, particularly those in authority. Such a system, if effective, will be flexible.

Let me repeat that such a process of change requires years, but a therapeutic culture, once established, can survive the changes of staff if new staff are more motivated to learn and grow. We are conceptualizing a system which has its own dynamic and promotes change in both patients and staff. Some people recognize a treatment modality loosely called social therapy, but I prefer to think of a social system for change which is complementary to other treatment methods, whether psychotherapeutic or organic. The term social learning seems more appropriate to me because the same concepts of systems theory apply to other social organizations such as schools, churches, factories, etc.

Discussion and Implications for Addictions Services

The term therapeutic community may be here to stay but, if so, the inevitable confusion might be lessened by adopting the term Programmatic Therapeutic Communities (P.T.C.) for the drug-free residential units and Democratic Therapeutic Communities (D.T.C.) for the mental health treatment model as suggested by Glaser (1983). For DTCs, we should change to a descriptive term like Democratic Change System (D.C.S.) and drop the term TC. However, psychiatrists might object, as DCS emphasizes Systems Theory and a Behavioral Science approach rather than "patients," doctors and psychotherapy, i.e., a medical approach.

From the point of view of social organization, I am somewhere in between the two extremes of PTCs and the doctor dominated medical model TCs. I see the position of the client or "patient" as more central in the total system of a PTC than in many DTCs where patients tend to project responsibility for treatment on the staff who assume this role all too readily. Patients and staff should share the responsibility as far as the patients' clinical condition permits.

Social learning in DTCs is essentially shared communication in a group setting where each individual learns to listen to other people's points of view and compare these with his own. Given interest and average intelligence, it is almost impossible not to absorb some new awareness of the topic under discussion. One's original viewpoint is thus modified. This is the learning process. It is enhanced when certain conditions are met, including: (a) regularly scheduled meetings, so that a learning process and growth can occur, over time; (b) staff who have psychodynamic skills both individual and group; (c) a high trust level in the group resulting from the group demonstrating its integrity, motivation, compassion, and confidentiality over time; (d) resulting from this is the security and freedom to communicate thoughts and feelings ("the truth") without fear of reprisal; (e) process reviews for staff training immediately following the daily community meeting as already described.

In such a group setting it usually becomes apparent that the group is more than the sum of the inputs of the individual members, and the individual tends to find his identity through the group. An important step for personality disorders who have usually been "losers" lacking a supportive peer group or even a clear identity. To me the existential procedures of PTCs insisting on personal responsibility to conform to a mandatory code of rules, and rewarded by a rise in status if successful, is a much narrower form of learning than the DTCs concept of social learning. The process of growth to a more mature individual is lacking, although as Deitch and Zweben (1983) point out ". . . the treatment of character and personality disorders, and some psychiatric disorders absolutely requires some coercive elements, to break down character defenses and promote the acquisition of impulse control." Some people may dislike the empirical method of "breaking down" defenses, but probably the majority of psychiatrists have, at one time or another, used electric convulsion therapy!

Despite the fundamentally different social organizations of DTCs and PTCs both have unusually strong and supportive social systems which effects the bonding essential to lasting change, and both are in sharp contrast to the relatively "distant" social environment found in most psychiatric residential facitities.

Leadership is viewed very differently by the two types of TC. The extraordinary authority and power invested in the position of leader in a PTC requires steps be taken to contain any abuse of power (O'Brien and Biase, 1981). My own position on this subject is viewed as extreme by many of my own profession and is described elsewhere (Jones, 1982). In brief, I believe in multiple leadership with distribution of responsibility and authority throughout the system. When I was the head of a mental hospital in Scotland, it took me 7 years to distribute the authority to wherever was deemed appropriate in the system and, thereby, did myself out of a job. I felt sad but rewarded!

Personally, I find much food for thought by comparing the two systems. We know so little about social systems for change, that both models justify careful study. The dichotomy between the autocratic and the democratic is familiar throughout history, and at the present time remains unanswered in politics, business, religion, and international relations, to mention only a few. Maybe the answer lies ultimately in some appropriate blend, as may well be the case with PTCs and DTCs.

CHAPTER 3

THE PSYCHODYNAMICS OF THEREAPEUTIC COMMUNITIES FOR TREATMENT OF HEROIN ADDICTS

MARTIEN KOOYMAN

T
HE EXISTING literature shows few positive results of individual psychotherapy applied in the treatment of heroin addicts. On the contrary, often heroin addiction is seen as a counter-indication for psychotherapy. Individual psychotherapy for addicts is generally seen as useless if the addict continues to use his drug. In view of the high relapse rate, as a condition, an abstinence period of at least half a year is necessary before individual psychotherapy can be effectively applied.

Different methods of group psychotherapy, however, are applied successfully in the treatment of heroin addicts, particularly group therapy with emphasis on direct confrontations of the behaviour in the "here and now" and on direct emotional interactions. Examples are psychodrama, encounter groups, scream therapy and groups stressing the importance of learning alternative ways of behaviour (assertive training, Transactional Analysis, reality therapy). (Siroka, 1971)

Non-psychotherapeutic groups such as self help groups are also an excellent tool for helping addicts to live a drug-free life. The self help concept was originally introduced by Alcoholic Anonymous (AA). The therapeutic communities (TCs) in the USA were developed from the self help concept. Histories of the development of therapeutic communities are available elsewhere and will not be repeated here.

After the second World War therapeutic communities for psychiatric patients were developed in several countries, following the model of Maxwell Jones (Jones, 1953). Jones's model, where the democratic atmosphere was an important component, was unsuccessful for addicts since it could not provide the necessary limits to their behaviour. Within those therapeutic communities, the behaviour of especially young drug addicts, who appeared as a new problem in the late 60s, could not be dealt with. Separate therapeutic communities for addicts were founded, setting clear limits to the behaviour of the residents with strict rules on the use of alcohol, drugs and violence. Most of these therapeutic communities applied the concepts and structure of the self help therapeutic communities developed in the USA. The European therapeutic communities were also influenced by new group therapies developed in the USA as well as by European psychotherapy (Kooyman, 1978).

The Life-Style of Drug Addicts and the Psychodynamics of Their Behaviour

The use of drugs by addicted persons can in most cases be seen as a symptom of underlying problems. The nature of these problems can be psychological, interpersonal and/or social. Psychological problems can vary from a character disorder to neurotic or psychotic disease. Drug abuse can be considered as a self-administered medicine to diminish feelings of tension or pain from a large variety of origin. There might exist a severe psychological disorder, such as schizophrenic or affective psychosis, a borderline syndrome, and so on. With a serious underlying psychiatric disorder, successful treatment in a regular therapeutic community for heroin addicts cannot be expected. The behaviour of such patients is too complicated for the staff and fellow-residents, so their admission usually results in rejection and expulsion from the therapeutic community (Lakoff, 1978).

Most residents of therapeutic communities belong to the character disorder type of heroin addicts. Because of this, the development of their behavioural pattern which may ultimately lead to heroin addiction will be described.

Prior to their first drug use, these addicts display a behaviour which serves as a protection against unconscious, painful feelings. The subsequent use of drugs helps them to attain the same goal (Whishnie, 1977). The addict is unable — and already was so before his drug abuse — to ask other people for help in a direct way. He controls the situation through manipulative behaviour, protecting himself against rejection. His behaviour is aimed at immediate gratification. Addicts have no trust in the future; they have a basic distrust of others as well as an absolute lack of self confidence. Contrary to common belief, addicts do not enjoy the pleasures of life. They fear success and tend to behave in a destructive manner. Almost all ex-addicts show extreme difficulties in getting in touch with the feeling that they have the right to exist. Bassin described heroin addicts as people who are, (due to a deeply rooted distrust of other people), unable to sustain meaningful relationships and also present a failure identity (Bassin, 1976).

The dependence on the effect of heroin and the involvement of the accompanying life-style can be seen as an adaptation to an impaired ego-development. Saari (1976) states that heroin addict of the character disorder type suffers from defects in the pre-genital development of the personality. Particularly in the separation/individuation stage, the period in which feelings of self-esteem, control of impulses and super-ego function are developed, a critical period can be found in the family situation. Usually the child received inconsistent messages and unclear limits were set to his behaviour; the parents were frequently absent and often there was a serious emotional deprivation. In this situation the child develops guilt feelings and thinks that he caused the loss of affection. As a result, painful effects are linked to feelings of hopelessness, being worthless and unlovable. Often an extreme separation anxiety develops in the absence of an internalization of positive object relations and an impaired super-ego development is unavoidable (Hollidge, 1980). The foundation is then set for a serious inhibition for separation from the parent's home in late adolescence. Use of drugs can meet the need for affection and support from a parent can be met immediately. Accompanying feelings of guilt are linked with the notion of not being entitled to good feelings and affection. The unavoidable misery linked to drug abuse is a symbolic solution for this internal conflict. The addict is as dependent on the positive experience of the drug use as on the accompanying misery. The most important defence mechanism is projection. All negative feelings of the addict are projected into others. His failure is caused by others. Society tries to take away the only identity he ever got: the identity of a junky.

A therapeutic community offers an environment that enables the heroin addict to free himself from his early pre-genital fixation. In this environment the drug addict can be helped to regain his feelings of self-esteem, to develop trust in others and to learn to separate from his new family in a healthy way.

External Factors Influencing the Individual's Development and Continuation of His Addiction

Dependence on drugs may be caused by a distrubance of the balance between the following factors: (1) outside pressure; (2) support from the environment; and (3) the autonomy of the individual (Uchtenhagen, 1981). When one of these factors dominates the others or if one of these factors is not sufficiently present, the individual experiences stress, which drugs can temporarily diminish. The addict found a surrogate solution for his problems. He feels good despite the threatening, boring or painful experience of personal, interpersonal or social origin. He got trapped in the vicious circles of the addiction: his only remaining problem is how to get the drug in order to feel good or just feel normal. Provided the drug is easily obtainable and its use does not cause additional problems such as a poor physical condition, lack of money, or the threat of being arrested, motivation to stop using the drug will generally not occur.

In most cases external factors lead to a decision to ask for help. We can consider the admission as a first necessary step to treatment, a step that is not easy to take. Stopping the use is only a first step into treatment. We can distinguish four vicious circles in which the addict is likely to be caught: (1) the pharmacological circle; (2) the psychological circle; (3) the environmental circle; and (4) the social vicious circle.

In general these circles have the following effect: discontinuation of the use causes an effect that is opposite to the desired effect of the drug; if the addict starts to use the drug again, this annoying, undesired effect disappears. This is the **pharmacological vicious circle**. The addict feels guilty because of his drug abuse. The unpleasant guilt feelings disappear when he uses the drug again. This is the **psychological vicious circle**.

In the immediate **environment** of the addict, his addiction serves as a function to sustain a pathological balance. This can be the case within a family: the child is the scape-goat. His abuse distracts the attention from existing problems within the family. If he stops his drug abuse, serious problems within the family can become apparent, and as a result the child re-assumes his role of the scape-goat and so restores the pathological balance within the family.

The social stigmatization of the addict seriously hinders his re-integration. It is difficult to convince people that once an addict doesn't mean always an addict. The addict feels only accepted by his fellow-users. This is the **social vicious circle**.

In the treatment of addicts, the pharmacological vicious circle is eliminated. The addict can no longer use his drug to prevent the unpleasant feelings re-appearing after stopping his abuse. During treatment the addict learns to step out of the psychological vicious circle by talking about his feelings of guilt rather than "bottle them up" with the use of drugs. The negative influence of the immediate environment is eliminated by offering a new environment: a therapeutic community.

Goals and Principals of a Therapeutic Community

The goal of treatment in a therapeutic community goes beyond the treatment of the individual's behaviour; this behaviour is considered as a symptom of underlying problems. Only after the use of drugs has stopped, do the problems appear. In a therapeutic community the individual is taught to regain feelings of trust in himself and in others. The final goal is not neutral, but positive. The resident of a therapeutic community is taught to deal with stress and conflicts in a constructive way. He is also taught that asking for help does not mean being helpless.

TC treatment aims at social, intellectual, physical and creative development of the resident. In this process it is important that the resident learns to discover the limits of his capacities, to learn that he is not the giant of his dreams, nor the dwarf of his fears and that this is okay.

A TC is defined as an environment where people stay together with a common goal, that is, to solve the problems they were unable to solve. To attain this, they try to construct consistent, and in itself logical patterns of collaboration, in which social learning can take place. The basic philosophy of self help therapeutic communities is that the residents learn to help themselves with the help of others. The program is obligatory and the same for everyone. Residents learn to express themselves in groups. There are strict house rules: no use of alcohol or drugs, no use of violence or threatening with violence; breaking these rules means immediate removal from the therapeutic community. Substitute drugs or psychotropic medicines are not used in treatment in a drug free TC.

An important element in the treatment is that the resident learns to make his life public; to share his secrets with others; to get to know himself; to get rid of his feelings of guilt and shame by talking about those feelings with others. The resident learns to respect important values in life, such as honesty, concern and responsibility. For this longer term residents serve as a role model for their newer fellows.

The Therapy

The therapy is the sum of everything that is happening in the TC. The whole program is directed to the ultimate goal. The structure offers safety and security for the resident. It also provides ample opportunities to practice assumed responsibilities at different levels (Bratter and Kooyman, 1980). Residents are stimulated to choose a constructive way of living.

Hollidge (1980) described the following curative elements existing in a therapeutic community:

1. **The Instilling of Hope.** Upon admission, the resident sometimes suffers from conscious feelings of hopelessness and worthlessness. He failed in everything, even as an addict. In a therapeutic community the resident is explained that he can change. Such a change is not possible without causing conflicts; if there is no conflict, there is no stimulus to change. It is very difficult to instill hope for a positive change in individual or in group therapy on a outpatient basis, since the client is re-inforced outside the sessions in his continuing failure. In the climate of a therapeutic community, where no-one is ever seen as hopeless and the person in question is stimualted to use his existing potential, it is possible to eliminate the feelings of hopelessness and worthlessness (Yalom, 1975).

2. **Feelings of Togetherness.** Confrontation with the problems of fellow-residents makes the resident's problems no longer unique. Recognition of the other's situation develops confidence and trust. Contrary to the situation in individual or group therapy the TC client does not feel alienated from social life.

3. **Altruism.** Most addicts believe that they are of no value to others. By helping others, their feelings of self-esteem are reinforced.

4. **Socialization.** Instead of the manipulative behaviour that the addict displayed to others in order to satisfy his own needs, the resident learns new communicative skills. He learns to ask for help in a direct way.

5. **Development of Interpersonal Skills and Sharing Information.** The residents learn to express and to accept criticism. Through exchanging experiences he gets the necessary insight into his own behaviour improving reality-testing.

6. **Group Cohesion.** New residents may see the TC as the bad object and consequently isolate themselves for fear of rejection. Confrontation of this gives insight into this behaviour. Feelings of belonging to the

group have to be developed in order to eliminate underlying feelings of not being accepted.

7. **Re-Living Situations From the Family of Origin**. A TC serves as a new family in which positive expectations can be experienced.

8. **Identification**. The first positive relationships with fellow-residents can create different identification from that toward parents. The old identity is left behind and positive introjections occur, producing an increase of self-esteem, insight and trust.

These elements are part of a larger therapeutic environment.

Therapeutic Tools

1. **Structure of the Program**. In the program residents learn to perform various social roles with different responsibilities. They learn to make errors without the feeling of being completely worthless and to explore their potentials and limitations. It is important to learn to show interest in other people and, by doing so, give up narcistic behaviors. Responsibilities are delegated to the residents as much as possible regarding the day-to-day management in the community.

2. **Encounter Groups**. The type of encounter group described here are the confrontation groups, developed from the Synanon game (Liebermann et. al., 1973). In almost all TCs for addicts this kind of group therapy is the most important therapeutic tool. Here everyday conflicts can be worked out to teach residents to express their irritations in a direct way and to deal with their emotions. The starting point is the "here-and-now" situation. If there is a link with situations from the past, these can be worked out in the "here-and-now." In these groups, expressing emotions by screaming is used to get in touch with feelings that have been depressed for a long time. A catharsis in itself, however, is not enough. Underlying attitudes are worked through, defining the behaviour in order to attain the necessary insight into oneself. During encounter groups the attention and concentration is focussed on one person at a time. This is called "group focus." The basic philosophy behind this confrontation is that criticism is okay. However, criticism should not be meant to hurt the other person. An encounter group is not a discussion group. The most important element is the learning from experience obtained in the group. In the group a person is encouraged to do just what he fears most in order to learn this by training. Although groups can be led by residents, usually one of the staff leads the group. During the groups, staff can also be confronted. During the group ses-

sions negotiation, identification and projection can occur. For a participant it is often more important what he himself says to others than what
is said to him: he confronts himself in the other person.

At the start of an encounter group, that lasts about two hours, irritations are usually ventilated. This can become a highly emotional situation. With feelings of helplessness, loneliness, pain and sorrow. In most
cases the groups end in a quiet atmosphere of mutual involvement. As a
contrast to the often heavy emotional confrontations, it is important to
allow humor in the group, to laugh at behaviour. At the end of a group
the participants give their feed-back to what happened in the group.

3. **Other Therapeutic Tools.** At different times in the program extended groups can be used, varying in length from one day (probes) to
groups that least several days with only limited periods to sleep
(marathons). These groups can devote themselves to certain themes,
such as unfinished business from the past, sexuality, intimacy, creativity,
plans for the future and so on.

An important form of group therapy, adapted in many TCs for addicts, are cathartic groups, also called scream groups or bonding groups,
developed by Casriel. Casriel himself calls it N.I.P. groups (New Identity Process) (Casriel, 1972). In these groups participants learn to deal
with intimacy and the accompanying emotions. Most important is to
work through the pathological attitudes that prevent the participant
from enjoying intimacy and pleasure.

In many TCs acting out behaviour is confronted in a clear way,
sometimes according to a fixed pattern. It can be a "haircut," a verbal
reprimand in which a person that has been misbehaving is talked to by
two or three peers. They point out to him the negative elements of his
behaviour, connecting it with his previous behaviour that ultimately
brought him into the community. The person in question is not allowed
to answer only think, since in many cases addicts are very good in defense roles.

The TC sets clear limits to negative, destructive behaviour. This behaviour is seen as avoiding direct emotional confrontations, for which
many possiblities are given in the encounter groups. Direct emotional
confrontations replace acting out behaviour here.

Sometimes a resident is told to exaggerate certain aspects of his pe-
sonality in order to increase his self knowledge. Therefore, it is not unusual to see someone moving through the TC dressed like a cowboy, a
nurse, a wise man or with an outfit reinforcing certain aspects of his behaviour.

In the TC structure the resident can have different positions with increasing responsibilities. The staff decides on the position of the resident in the structure of the different departments. If, for example, somebody is in charge of the kitchen and is in that role able to provide good meals but does not notice that members of his crew are considering to use drugs again, it may be made clear to him that he'd better work in the crew again to learn where they, collectively stand.

The Therapeutic Community as a Socio-Educative Instrument

The TC is not only a psychotherapeutic instrument. An important aspect of TC life is learning to interact with others and to deal with interpersonal conflicts; "social learning through social interaction" (Jones, 1953).

In a TC a crisis is an important learning moment. During their stay in the therapeutic community, residents often discover new possibilities to express themselves in a creative way and upgrading school knowledge is another part of the program. Residents sometimes have to relearn what learning means. This is very important for residents who intend to go back to school again.

The Therapeutic Process

If the resident can no longer hide his problem by using drugs or alcohol, if he can no longer use violence and if it is almost impossible to withdraw from the group, feelings of irritation, fear and anger, pain and despair may appear.

As in all psychotherapeutic situations, the resident initially raises his defenses. This behaviour is accepted and seen as a necessary step towards growing up again in the proper way. Acting out behaviour appears, and for which limits are clearly set. Since there is a quick response to acting out behaviour, real severe disasters such as serious physical violence or suicidal attempts very rarely occur. Before someone actually develops such behaviour, attention has already been paid to this destructive behaviour on a smaller scale. Very often regression takes place. Infantile feelings from the family of origin are transferred to members of the new family. Transfer and counter transfer takes place. During the group sessions, the group leaders do not try to hide their counter transferences but express and discuss them. During regression, the resident becomes attached to the community and forms a personal identification with the group. By imitating older resident-role models, new behaviour is learned.

In the group clients learn to do those things they are most afraid of and learn to change the negative picture they hold of themselves. Many residents have to learn to feel that it is a pleasure to exist. From this awareness they learn to approach other people and to ask for help, to show emotion, to be vulnerable, and finally to learn to love themselves and others. They learn to take responsibilities, to deal with success, and to sustain relationships with others.

During the last phase of their stay residents seek their own identity. In this process they rebel, reject the values and norms of the TC as if they were adolescents again. At that time the resident is already in the re-entry phase of the program.

Different Phases in the Treatment

The TC program has several phases. Before admission there is an orientation or induction period, enabling the prospective client to make a clear decision to become an active member. During the first phase of the resident's stay development of trust is a primary goal. In most cases the resident trusts only one member of the community. Gradually he begins to trust more fellow-residents and finally the staff. The clear rules offer the resident (who frequently lacks a feeling of basic security and who has a deeply rooted distrust in human relationships) support and safety.

During the first month the new resident has to get accustomed to order and regularity. He will be confronted with his behaviour and his attitude. Later, attention will be focused on the way he relates to his fellow-residents.

The most critical period is when the resident gives up his defense that keeps him at a safe distance from the others. He feels insecure and vulnerable. If sufficient trust in the group has developed, the focus is on underlying emotional problems. This is the second phase. In this phase, the situation is reversed: the resident, previously confronted by others with his behaviour, now begins to confront others. He has found his place and is able to take responsibilities. The resident acquires a growing feeling of entitlement as he experiences to be of value to someone else.

During the third phase, treatment is directed particularly in preparing the resident for his stay in the re-entry program. An important aspect in this period is the development of relations outside the TC. At the same time the resident has become a role model for new residents in this phase.

The last phase of treatment is the re-entry program. This program can be located in a separate part of the TC or in a separate house. The latter is usually the case if the therapeutic community itself is located in the country and too far away from the town or city where re-entry into society has to take place. Separate peer groups are held for residents in the different phases of the program, focusing on the above mentioned areas.

The Re-Entry Program

In the re-entry program the separation from the program takes place; for most residents a difficult process. Staff has to be aware of the important role of separation problems. It is important that staff is not trapped into paying attention only to the negative side of the resident's behaviour. There is a real danger that residents live up to negative expectations in an unconscious way, especially if this occurs as a repetition of the negative expectations of their parents.

It is also possible that staff may have greater expectations than the residents can fulfill (Vos, 1983). In this phase of the program it is important that staff allows the resident to express criticism towards the treatment program. If criticism is not expressed directly, it may appear in the way of acting out behaviour such as smoking marijuana, abusing alcohol, not keeping appointments and so on. It is important to have regular group meetings of re-entry residents, allowing them to express their criticism.

Negative behaviour is part of the separation process. Often these problems go back to the separation problems of the parental home. The emotional process of separation can only occur if the resident has gained enough emotional distance from the program. While individual therapy is not generally applied it definitely has its place in the re-entry program. Individual sessions with the resident may take place in addition to the re-entry groups. Re-occuring destructive behaviour can be considered as a denial of the reality of an earlier rejection by the parents. Insight into the behaviour can be gained in the individual sessions in the re-entry program. It appears that many residents have maintained the fantasy that they are worthless and the cause of all problems. Only if sufficient trust in the therapist and the experience in the therapeutic community has given the resident enough ego-strength, successful individual psychotherapy can be applied in the re-entry program.

Usually the re-entry program is completed after about one year.

During the last months of the program the client lives on his own and contacts with the program are limited to occasional participation in groups and individual consultations at the client's request.

Treatment Results

Addicts are notorious for dropping out of treatment soon after their admission (e.g., De Leon and Schwartz, 1984). Only if the negative motivation has changed into a positive one (in some cases this only happens after a stay of several months) treatment may be expected to be successful.

Currently, a follow-up research is being carried out among the first 250 ex-residents of the Emiliehoeve therapeutic community (Kooyman, 1975). Ex-residents are interviewed after their departure. If no relapse into their addiction has occurred, they are then followed-up during a period of 5 years with at least two more interviews. The preliminary results of this study show that residents who stay longer in the program are less likely to relapse into their addiction. The results give an indication that treatment for those who followed the program is worth the effort.

Application of the Model of a Therapeutic Community for Addicts for Other Categories of Residents

A TC for addicts distinguishes itself from TCs developed in Europe for the treatment of psychiatric patients according to the principles of Maxwell Jones. Acting-out behaviour is immediately confronted, preventing it from becoming an unmanageable situation. Because of this, the TCs for addicts are also suitable for patients with severe "acting-out" tendencies, for example, hysterical and suicidal behaviour, patients with automutulation, anorexia nervosa and so on. It is worthwhile to try this treatment modality for a larger scope of potential residents who are treated in psychiatric centers (Jongsma, 1980) and for juvenile delinquents.

Summary and Conclusion

The deeply rooted lack of trust of drug addicts in others and the connecting manipulative behaviour make them largely unsuitable for traditional forms of psychotherapy, especially for individual psychotherapy. A TC for addicts offers an environment in which trust in other people can develop gradually, enabling the resident to regain trust in himself. In the TC the resident learns to change acting out behaviour into direct emotional confrontation, also learning to solve conflicts and critical situations once avoided. Follow-up research shows that ex-residents are able to function well outside the safety of the TC without returning to their old addictive behaviour.

Drug addiction and the related acting out behaviour protects the person from experiencing pain and fear from a variety of origins. Most drug addicts, however, show a defect in their ego-development, especially during the separtation/individuation phase. This results in the development of a failure identity with projection as the main defense mechanism. The addict shows a serious lack of self-esteem and a considerable distrust in other people, who are usually seen as a potential source of pain. In the structured environment of the TC the lack of trust in others can be restored gradually.

CHAPTER 4

BRITAIN AND THE PSYCHOANALYTIC TRADITION IN THERAPEUTIC COMMUNITIES

ROBERT D. HINSHELWOOD

B EING from Britain, this article may appear somewhat insular. However, there is more than a geographical divide. Therapeutic communities in Britain and America are separated by a conceptual and historical divide as well.

In Britain the therapeutic community has an extended history going back to the beginnings of this century and before. A significant precursor was the work of an American who set up an experiment in progressive education in Britain in 1913. This was Homer Lane who was appointed to run the Little Commonwealth (Wills, 1964). But the project itself was initiated in Britain and stands firmly in the nineteenth century tradition of founding small, discrete utopian groups living together according to ideals and principles that were quite consciously opposed to the values of developing industrial society.

Independently of this and other precursors, the therapeutic community really first happened in a military hospital in England in 1941. There were a number of attempts, in fact, in the same hospital during the war years. The first was set up by W.R. Bion (Bion & Rickman, 1943). He was a veteran of the First World War, who commanded the first, and I believe the only, tank battle of that war. Whatever happened to his tanks I don't know but at Northfield he lost and was sacked after six weeks because he would not take responsibility from his patients for the mess they had made:

"Faced with a ward full of neurotic soldiers . . . slovenly, undisciplined, idle and dirty . . . Bion had viewed their behaviour . . . as a collusion . . .

43

where the staff are to be well and self-disciplined and patients are to be ill and disordered. He told his patients at a daily ward parade that he was fed up with them, and henceforth refused to be responsibile for caring about, treating or disciplining delinquent behaviour which was theirs and not his. He would not punish them. . . He would be available for discussion in his office every morning but only for soldiers who presented themselves clean and properly dressed. In the next weeks they severely tested out his resolve. . . It was chaotic, but Bion plainly did not get his DSO in the First World War for nothing. . . Bion's ward became the most efficient in the hospital. This was a bold imaginitive innovative experiment . . . in the delegation of health and responsibility to patients" (Main, 1977).

Though a short-lived failure it clearly made a deep impression and has led many to write about it —

"a 'leaderless' ward system was set up which was designed to display neurosis in the individual, primarily not for the patient and the medical staff but as a problem for the whole group, in this instance the ward. . . The problem of bed-wetting, for instance, was not left to be coped with in the secretive orthodox way by the nursing staff, which increased the soldiers' sense of disgrace and inadequacy, but as a problem for the whole ward which had to be discussed openly at the ward meetings. . . Bion and Rickman participated as observers. The prime reason for terminating the experiment lay in the anxiety of the 'authorities' that such a radical approach would undermine discipline and the last straw came when the dining-hall was left in a state of disorder following a film-show and the floor was left strewn with newspapers and used contraceptives" (deMare, 1983).

Then came Tom Main who on observing Bion's defeat took a wider view of therapy —

"Bion had been therapeutic for his ward but anti-therapeutic for the military staff, successful in his ward . . . but highly disturbing to the hospital" (Main, 1977).

Out of this conception of the whole institution of the hospital (the patients and also the staff) Main produced the concept of an institution that could itself be therapeutic — he coined the term therapeutic community (Main, 1946).

Many others contributed to these experiments at Northfield. We should not perhaps forget the major contribution made by Hitler himself! He mobilized whole groups or communities and was a vivid example for the whole of Europe! And the idea of dealing with a social entity became very prevalent in Churchill's Britain because of the mobilization of the army and of the whole country to fight a war. At the same time German academic life had been dispersed, including the highly influential gestalt psychologists. Applied to groups, gestalt psychology came to

Britain just before the war via America as Kurt Lewin's field theory of groups (Lewin, 1936); and directly, through S.H. Folkes (1948) who also began at Northfield.

Thus there were many sources in the prehistory of the therapeutic community in Britain. Kennard (1983), in his extraordinarily careful dissection of the numerous historical roots, describes some eight or so formative factors. The Northfield group of psychiatrists were largely psychoanalysts, and the British version of the therapeutic community bears the marks of this history. So, as well as the medial model of professional therapy, and the dominating idea of mobilizing social entities, there was a major input from the theory and practice of psychoanalysis.

After the war this mixture blended with other principles of pre-therapeutic communities — the humanity of progressive education and the utopianism of religious communities. Later, in the 1960's, with the surge towards democracy, permissiveness and revolution, the therapeutic community movement acquired a radical political dimension, often known as anti-psychiatry (Laing, 1960; Cooper, 1967), which related uncomfortably to the professional medical founding fathers.

This melange has bubbled away for decades, provoking the sober, scientific, psychiatric institutions. So when, around 1970, an American version of therapeutic communities appeared in Britain and Europe, we thought we could absorb this curiosity. But, like Mohammedaus all facing Mecca to pray, the American devoutly faced Synanon. And, disconcertingly, they had not the slightest interest in the hectic free-for-all of the British therapeutic community movement. These oddities took on a sinister quality when their disciplinary activities became known — why had Europe torn its own heart out to get rid of fascism, only to be invaded by transatlantic, brainwashing, concentration camps of this kind!

Well, a decade later some of the mists have cleared and British and American therapeutic communities are making a more cautious appraisal of each other (for example Almond, 1974; Glaser, 1983; Sugarman, 1984). The rest of this paper will look out from my own psychoanalytically-based experience of British therapeutic communities.

Looking From a Psychoanalytic Perspective

The British version of therapeutic communities owes a major dept to psychoanalysts who tried to use their framework to understand and

work with social systems. It is not just the group therapy traditions
started by Foulkes and Bion, or the therapeutic community developed
over the years by Tom Main at the Cassel hospital, but Bion, Rice, Trist
and others have developed human relations training (Rice, 1965; see
also Turquet, 1975), and the Tavistock Institute of Human Relations
has developed methods of organization development (Jaques, 1951;
Menzies, 1960; Miller & Gywnne, 1972; see also the reviews by Sofer,
1972; and deBoard, 1978).

However, this is a tradition that over the years has moved aside from
the mainstream of therapeutic communities. Old-fashioned psychoanalytic concepts of 80 years ago have been retained as the therapeutic community embraced many other concepts (Jones, 1952; Rapoport, 1960;
Clark, 1964; Whiteley, Briggs & Turner, 1972).

When, in 1955, Rapoport and his team of social anthroplogists went
into The Henderson Hospital at Maxwell Jones's invitation, their results
were interesting. They discovered four principles which the community
tried to work to. These principles had not been explicitly worked out by
the staff but had developed intuitively. It was only with outside researchers that they could be singled out and formalized as the great hallmarks
of the British therapeutic community. The work of defining these principles promoted a clear identity for the therapeutic community in Britain.
Otherwise it would have slid into vagueness, discredit and oblivion like
the milieu therapy movement in America in the 1950s.

The four principles formulated by Rapoport were: communalism,
democratization, permissiveness and reality-confrontation (Rapoport,
1960). Although Jones's work at the Henderson had turned away from
psychoanalysis, the principles bore a remarkable imprint of their psychoanalytic paternity. Permissiveness and reality-confrontation corre-
spond in the social setting to the free association and interpretation of
psychoanalytic practice.

Psychoanalysis has developed too (somewhat differently in Britain
compared to American). Major changes in theory and practice have
taken place which could allow the newer psychoanalysis, particularly the
ideas of Klein (Segal, 1964) (splitting, projection and introjection) to
bear in new ways on the therapeutic community. These concepts
describe the way in which experiences and feelings can be defensively
disowned, or recovered in the social context. My own involvement has
been to work out applications to therapeutic communities (Hinshelwood, 1979).

The Cultures

Much has been written of the permissiveness of British communities (Zeitlyn, 1967; Morrice, 1979), especially during the "political" phase during the 1960s. In practice all that dust has settled. A community permits action and relationships within a set of limits which (a) are clear; and (b) are as broadly stretched as is compatible with reasonably good order. In most forms of psychotherapy and psychoanalysis the limits are drawn to permit any verbal behaviour, but to exclude all activity that is not verbal. It is called free association. In a community, people live and act together on all sorts of tasks. So the idea of free association is extended to the way people relate to each other and the way they organize and function within the organization they create. The creative action then forms the basis for confronting the person with the reality he lives in, by showing him the reality he has created.

Within limits then, the British communities "run free." We can say, therefore, that no two communities are alike. And no one community stays the same for very long. There is no obvious prototype. This is true in a sense. But where they do conform is in their approach to variation.

They note it, where it comes from and who contributes to it.

Morale goes up and down. There are phases of certain kinds of acting out — going absent, rows and fights, mutism, use of alcohol, idealization of an individual (staff or patient), fashionable interests in a particular part of the program. The mood of the community and the community meetings varies — depressed, sulky, compliant, active, controlling, over-confident.

How an individual contributes, is what he learns about himself. The community has an important task in analyzing its own culture. That is, it is there to find a meaning for the individuals in the variation and the current relationships of the community.

The common culture of British communities is that they are "cultures for analysis."

The American version of therapeutic communities has not had the same romance with psychoanalysis. These are derived from a behavioral or re-educative model.

The culture of the American version is radically different. It is homogeneous, and little Synanons have sprung up the world over as a series of identical clones. The cultural and structural uniformity is impressive. What is this resilient and self-reproducing culture?

Dederich, quoted by Yablonsky (1965), described the climate of Synanon as —

> "A more or less autocratic family structure . . . used to administer doses of an inner-directed philosophy such as that outlined in Emmerson's essay entitled Self Reliance." He acknowledges it may be "paradoxical that an authoritative environment tends to produce inner direction."

Residents are taught concepts which explain their problems. They are expected to take on board "a complete handbook of behaviour, attitudes, and values" (Kennard, 1983). Central to this are the addicts' problems of sporting an image in defiance of his true nature, propped up by his dress, "street-talk" and the high from his drugs. Therapy, based on the encounter group rationale, requires "the cracking of facades" as Rogers (1969) puts it and this may have to be done very violently.

My exposure to the American version has been from visits and extensive discussions with people who have resided there. I have always come away impressed with the sense of energy and belief. For those who stick with the program, the "teaching" certainly goes in. The incessant onslaught on the residents' personalities bares them. To rebuild they have only the "force fed" concepts of the community and their own raw and naked feelings.

The theory then is that this new "inner-directed" attitude is the foundation of self-reliance.

Responsibility as a Pivotal Concept

Responsibility is a pivotal concept in both versions of therapeutic communities.

Often couched in the phrase "being responsible for oneself and one's feelings," the culture of the American version is a 24-hour infusion (recall Dederich's word "dose") of responsibility that the residents are expected to assimilate into their personalities. It is a responsibility to the others of the community, but a responsibility for what he truly is and how he truly feels. It is a responsibility to be honest and open with others, and about them, and to care for them, and for the community's behaviour, attitudes and values.

Success in the community means rising to positions of greater responsibility — real responsibility for the community, and very real penalties for failing.

In thinking about the British version, in the terms of the American one, I have been increasingly struck by the way in which issues also seem to orbit continually around problems of responsibility. Let me describe a short example.

> The community led itself astray as happens with permissive limits. But the waywordness allowed a view into various undercurrents. This community was a program for day attenders but there was an associated small inpatient unit for patients to live in during critical phases in their treatment. Danny was a 25 year old man, depressed and lethargic. He came to the attention of the community for presistent oversleeping and being too late for the obligatory morning meeting. Unusually for this community which viewed symptoms from a psychoanalytic point of view, Danny's problem was defined as a bad habit which must be broken. This was tackled by a community decision to admit Danny to the inpatient unit where his sleeping and working could be formed into new habits. This failed; because although he woke at the right time while sleeping in the hospital, he resumed his old pattern immediately after he left. Interestingly he was himself considerably concerned that such expensive treatment (full-time nursing care for which he did not have to pay the National Health Service) should be expended on him for the simple task of breaking his habit. And then he was especially concerned when it was a wasted expense.
>
> In fact it subsequently became clear from a psychoanalytic point of view that his oversleeping was an actively motivated symptom and not just a habit. It had a meaning in the totality of his life. His guilt and inadequacy over wasting the hospital resources was linked with his waste of his university education (he has never taken his finals) which his working class family had put such a high value on — higher than their son's happiness, so he believed.
>
> The point of the example is that the way in which this man's problem was formulated, took away his own responsibility for it. It was a habit and he should not have to feel the guilt of his own motivation. This was at a time when there had been a good deal of absenteeism and destructive waste of time by a number of people in the community. So there was general investment in evading guilt.
>
> Interestingly the staff too were caught up in this lapse. At this time there were questions from the administration about the use and effectiveness of the inpatient unit.

This kind of approach allows us to understand the collective defensiveness in the whole community though it gets caught up in just one person's case. Thus the community can lapse for a moment from the program described above as "delegating health and responsibility to the patient." And through understanding the lapse we gain access to a lot of things going on.

The evasion of responsibility be patients and the necessary return of it seems to me the fundamental dynamic flux of the British version of therapeutic communities. In their own ways both versions have this in common.

The Meaning of Responsibility

Without going into technicalities here, hesitant steps to and from responsibility and guilt, are a major feature of the Kleinian psychoanalytic view of maturation and therapy.

Responsibility means different things to different people. Perhaps one could put it that different kinds of people experience responsibility differently.

Some people find it cripplingly onerous and subsist in despair and depression. Others find it in a long-term satisfaction. There are those who constantly make others responsible. Slightly differently, some people have a peculiar habit of getting into situations in which someone else is continually telling them their responsibility. Above all there are some who appear to discount any responsibility at all.

These varieties of meaning are open to psychoanalytic understanding, which justifies the approach.

The Problem of Introjection

So some people lack an effective sense of responsibility. It is distorted, complex, maladaptive or missing. The approach of the British therapeutic community is to ask why, or where has it gone and why.

Not so in the American therapeutic community. There the approach to those who lack an adequate sense of responsibility is to set out to plant one vigorously in the heart of the resident. Questioning is circumvented by having a ready-made answer, already assumed in the culture. The answer is that responsibility is missing and has to be planted. The reasons why it is missing could be various, but the answer is always the same.

The way of achieving this is always the same, too — a dose of the culture, its concepts, its attitudes and its values.

The British therapeutic community would approach the problem by saying that the resident has a particular difficulty in taking something into himself, taking a sense of responsibility into his personality, keeping it safe and in working order. This is a problem of introjection.

Introjection is a psychological incorporation into the personality, equivalent to physical feeding. Difficulties that might prevent a sense of responsibility being incorporated are varied.

Again there would be the search for a meaning. The incorporation may be felt as though some poison is being administered so it is spat out. Or it may be felt as an intrusion from someone else, so like a rape it is resisted. Sometimes it seems as though there is no way to keep things inside and it, like everything else, leaks out like vomit/tears/diarrhea. Or else it may be felt that it is immediately wasted, by chewing over, and thus turned straight away into feces. And there are variations, combinations and alternatives to these phantasies.

The similarity between psychological and bodily happenings is, no doubt, apparent. It is these kinds of meanings that contemporary British psychoanalysts believe are close to the "bedrock" of personality; and of personal individuality. They would appear to lie somewhere near to where the mind merges with the body.

It is not my intention here to pursue the benefits to which these ideas can be put in the British therapeutic community. I shall merely use them in a comparable analysis of the culture of the American therapeutic community.

The Addictive Culture

The kinds of "bedrock" phantasies just described are not attended to in American therapeutic communities. And there may be a good reason why they do not need attention there.

Selection for those communities produces residents who are very uniform in two essential respects. They are all drug addicts who have given up their addiction; and they have all survived the early dropout stage of the program.

There may in fact be different types of drug addiction. Glover (1939) has already distinguished three psychoanalytic diagnoses in the drug addiction.

We are then led to a hypothesis: the selective process results in a group of residents who have remarkably similar "bedrock" phantasies.

What phantasy underlies this group of personalities? It is a curious one akin to those mentioned in the last section but with a modification. In their unconscious view they avidly incorporate poisons but triumphantly seek it and survive it (see for instance the review by Rosenfeld, 1964).

A therapeutic community that takes in a very selected group of residents who have similar "bedrock" phantasies is likely to generate a highly consistent culture. The culture will express something of the phantasy. If the "bedrock" phantasy concerns problems of introjection, then the culture of the community may develop features representing the processes of introjection and incorporation. I would suggest that the culture of the American therapeutic community does indeed show this. The concentration on inner-directedness, and the highly energized activity devoted towards injecting the culture into the residents, are cultural representations of the special phantasy I have described. The culture represents an addiction to the incorporation of a poisonous substance — i.e., responsibility.

As we are dealing with the level of personality where the body and the mind are not significanly distinguished, the sense of responsibility, which is often painful, is easily substituted for the phantasy of an actually damaging bodily poison.

The culture of the American therapeutic community is peculiarly adapted to represent a common personal disturbance in the unconscious life of the peculiarly consistent personalities of the residents.

As some support for my intricate hypothesis, I shall draw attention to a recent paper which also demonstrated this connection from body to mind, and from mind to social culture. DeJong (1983) described a similar occurrence of culture changing to represent personal phantasies en masse. It happens again to concern problems of incorporation, this time eating. The membership of his community accumulated more people with eating problems. The culture changed radically coming to represent the pattern of the individual sufferer of "so called" anorexia nervosa —

> "the eating habits slowly lost any unity of place, time and action. Precisely this happens to be the case in the pathological eating patterns of an anorexia nervosa patient . . . (and) the staff were like the parents of an anorexia patients" (DeJong, 1983).

The adaption of a culture to represent the common features of the members is an exceedingly important general observation of groups and communities. It remains to be explained.

If my explanations appear to be extraordinarily fanciful, it is because as a psychoanalyst I am concerned with the extraordinary phantasies that unconsciously cripple some peoples' lives.

Consequences

The British and American versions of therapeutic communities show striking differences, and also some similarities. The surface appearances could be compared but the main point of this paper is that they are better compared at a deeper level — particularly in relation to personal and unconscious phantasies about responsibility. Responsibility is a feature of communal life — all kinds. It is responsibility for one's personal bearing in public.

The two versions of the therapeutic community deal with responsibility in their own ways. The British version takes a questioning attitude to why it is so, with the chance of a more normative position growing. The American injects the norm. The thesis of this paper is that whereas the British version is therefore able to embrace a variety of disturbed forms of responsibility, the American version is very restrictive and can only respond to one kind of personality. That personality is one who has an excited experience of taking into himself something that he believes his unconscious phantasies to be damaging or poisonous.

If this thesis appears to be worth taking seriously, there are some important questions which arise and concern the effectiveness of the American therapeutic community for addicts.

1. Is the substitution of a psychological poison for a physical poison a genuine long-term solution?
2. If responsibility can be substituted for a bodily poison, what is done to "detoxify" it?
3. Does the community program actually change this addiction to pain or harm?
4. If poisons are regarded as exhilarating rather than threatening, what is done to modify that?
5. Do large numbers of people drop out because they do not share the standard "bedrock" phantasy?
6. Are there other standard "bedrock" phantasies that mark other circumscribed groups of addicts, for whom other kinds of therapeutic community culture could be designed (more wittingly)?
7. How could such non-standard phantasies be elucidated in these communities?
8. Could British therapeutic communities learn to use standard cultures for uniform phantasisers?

CHAPTER 5

THE THERAPEUTIC COMMUNITY: A CODIFIED CONCEPT FOR TRAINING AND UPGRADING STAFF MEMBERS WORKING IN A RESIDENTIAL SETTING

DAVID H. KERR

THIS PAPER describes the development of the therapeutic community certification manual and the central principles and concepts of a TC.

History

While the Therapeutic Community (TC) has pre-Christian origins (Hobart Mowrer, **Integrity Group**, 1968), I will be talking about the TC's development over the last 45 years. The TC concept evolved from a combination of alcoholics anonymous and the work of Maxwell Jones, Chuck Dederich and literally hundreds of others who integrated this common sense self-help therapy into a working, separate therapeutic modality especially effective with drug addicts and alcoholics. The concepts of self-help, no we-they dichotomy (or a flattened hierarchy), and positive peer pressure were introduced by the proponents of alcoholics anonymous and particularly Chuck Dederich in 1958 with his founding of Synanon.

Although most psychiatrists had given up any attempt to help the drug addict or alcoholic, Maxwell Jones persisted in similar work with mental patients at Dingleton Hospital in England. Jones realized that the hierarchy of traditional psychiatric mental hospitals had to be flattened, and in the 1940s he established group therapy based on individuals taking a major role in helping themselves and each other. Jones felt that there was

much to be learned from the entire environment in addition to the therapeutic sessions. The concept of social learning was introduced as the essence of the "therapeutic community." When Casriel and Yablonsky
studied the Synanon phenomena, they identified a similar TC process
naming it after Jones's initial model. Although Synanon evolved independently of Jones's work, the two concepts have many similarities and
dramatic differences.

Synanon spawned hundreds of TCs. Most differ from Synanon in
that they made efforts to reintegrate residents or members back into society while avoiding the cultish aspects of the Synanon community. In
some cases the effectiveness of the TC concept was overrated, especially
during the Sixties. It was and still is having a dramatic impact on
thousands of men and women who are drug or alcohol abusers.

As a result of outside pressures, especially by federal and local funding sources, TCs banded together in 1975 to create the Therapeutic
Communities of America (TCA). This group developed a Credentialing
and Accreditation Task Force to further codify and define the TC so
practitioners would have a more uniform concept for staff training and
staff development.

Hundreds of persons in America and Europe took part in a massive
information sharing effort primarily through correspondence and
dozens of drafts that eventually distilled the TC concepts into ten basic
parameters or competences. The word "competence" was adopted since
the codification was now being directed in the form of establishing minimum standards for TC line staff who would then be certified by the
Board of Directors of the Therapeutic Communities of America. The
following lists these ten competences as described in the TC manual:

1. Understanding and promoting self-help and mutual help.
2. Understanding and practicing positive role modeling.
3. Understanding of social learning versus didactic learning.
4. Understanding and promoting the concept of "no we-they dichotomy."
5. Understanding and promoting upward mobility and the privilege
   system.
6. Understanding and practicing the concept of "acting as if."
7. Understanding the relationship between belonging and individuality.
8. Understanding the need for a belief system within the community.

9. Ability to maintain accurate records.

10. Understanding and facilitating group process.

In researching certification efforts countrywide, the Therapeutic Community Credentialing and Accreditation Task Force was directed to create a specific TC certification manual. George Zeiner at NIDA suggested not developing a generic counseling certification model, but a specific competency based "recognition model" for TC counselors or coordinators.

The Therapeutic Community Certification Manual, therefore, is a manual specific to the field which defines the TC as a model of therapy different from the educational model, rehabilitation model, medical model, vocational model, or other models.

The definition of the TC was derived after several years of discussion and exchange and was adopted by Therapeutic Communities of America in 1979 and by the World Federation of Therapeutic Communities in 1981. The following is the definition:

"The primary goal of a Therapeutic Community (TC) is to foster personal growth. This is accomplished by changing an individual's life style through a community of concerned people working together to help themselves and each other.

"The Therapeutic Community represents a highly structured environment with defined boundries, both moral and ethical. It employs community imposed sanctions and penalities as well as earned advancement of status and privileges as part of the recovery and growth process. Being part of something greater than oneself is an especially important factor in facilitating positive growth.

"People in a Therapeutic Community are members, as in any family setting, not patients, as in an institution. These members play a significant role in managing the TC and acting as positive role models for others to emulate.

"Members and staff act as facilitators, emphasizing personal responsibility for one's own life and for self-improvement. The members are supported by staff as well as being serviced by staff, and there is a sharing of meaningful labor so that there is a true investment in the community, sometimes for the purpose of the survival.

"Peer pressure is often the catalyst that converts criticism and personal insight into positive change. High expectations and high commitment from both members and staff support this positive change. Insight into one's problems is gained through group and individual interaction, but learning through experience, failing and succeeding and experiencing the consequences, is considered to be the most potent influence toward achieving lasting change.

"The TC emphasizes the integration of an individual within this Community and the progress is measured within the context of that Community against the Community's expectations. It is this Community, along with the individual, that accomplishes the process of positive change in the member. The tension created between the individual and this Community eventually resolves in favor of the individual, and this transition is taken as an important measure of readiness to move toward integration into the larger society.

"Authority is both horizontal and vertical, encouraging the concept of sharing responsibility, and supporting the process of participating in decision making when this is feasible and consistent with the philosophy and objectives to the Therapeutic Community."

The manual carefully defines the ten competencies exemplifying each with behavioral vignettes. The manual offers a **code of ethics** and **bill of rights**. TCA encourages the use of the manual and the newly developed training tape as a staff development tool for all TC programs.

Discussion of the Therapeutic Community Concepts

While the definition is fairly self-explanatory, some areas bear emphasizing. One of the most important aspects of the TC is the concept of **self-help and mutual help**. In most residential institutions clients, patients or members exist individually and their only requirement is to be a good patient and to do as the doctors, nurses or therapists dictate. Traditionally, the phenomenon of institutionalization takes place for long-termers where clients or members learn to adapt to the expectations of the orderlies, nurses or staff by politely accepting their medication, responding appropriately, dressing accordingly, etc. The TC is not immune to this institutionalization process, but the injection of the concept of self-help and mutual help adds a whole new dimension. Members cannot retreat, nor can they expect a doctor to bring them the magic pill or cure. The TC expects all members to help themselves and to help each other towards specific goals of personal growth. Members are not allowed to "slip and slide" (regress). The only acceptable behavior is adopting an attitude of helpfulness to each other and themselves. This **mutual concern** and more **loving atmosphere** is evident in a TC and differentiating it from traditional institutions where there is a quiet, almost morose atmosphere.

Another aspect of the TC which is equally important is the concept of **ethics and members' rights**. Here the TC, as defined and described in the Certification Manual, is different from self-style cults such as Synanon where there are few ethical, moral or legal boundaries to guide the thinking and behavior of the staff and members. In the traditional, charismatic cult when the leader has an idea that he/she wants to inflict on the community, there is nothing stopping this: no code of ethics, no bill of rights, no objective board of directors, no grievance procedure. The TC must be differentiated from the many cults that may be similar in appearance.

Earned advancement and legitimate success are equally important aspects of the TC. With individual rights permeating institutions, the equally important concept of personal responsibilities to self and others is often ignored or minimized. The TC highlights the concept of personal responsibility and creates a structure for individuals to advance only through earned achievements. These achievements and privileges are more appreciated. The members learn of the small apsects of life that they previously took for granted. A good example of this is the responsibility that members have for the survival of their own community which includes making their beds, cleaning the rooms, maintaining the facility, servicing vehicles, cooking their food, procuring donations of food and other items, maintaining their own files (with staff input), as appropriate, etc. As members perform these basic functions, showing concern for each other as well as showing their own personal growth, they obtain advancement within the TC structure, usually in some form of recognized rank or status. This is strong reinforcement and is found to be highly contributory toward improved self-esteem and personal confidence.

As mentioned in the definition, TC people are called **"members" rather than "clients" or "patients."** Self-improvement and personal growth are active processes of self-help and mutual help. The traditional connotation of a patient or even client is an individual who receives help and gets better because of it. In a TC members seek help from themselves and from others. These others may be other members or staff members. Much of the growth in the TC is a result of the members' influence on each other in addition to a staff's role in facilitating personal growth. The term "member" is more natural when you speak of family members or community members. You do not speak of family "clients" or family "patients" or community "clients."

The **pressure of peers** is ongoing in any institutional setting. In prisons, there is the well known inmate network where you do not "rat" on other inmates and there is always the perpetuation of inmates against the "hacks," or correctional officers. This negative peer pressure in prisons often turns first offenders into hardened criminals. The TC turns this peer pressure around, creating the dynamic of positive peer pressure. Negative "tips" are broken up and positive peer pressure and **individual confessions** are strongly encouraged. Members must "rat on" each other in order for a TC to work. There are just not enough staff members to look around the community 24 hours a day and listen for "bad rapping," plotting, or negative or self-destructive discussion. The TC's role is not to stifle these discussions (this would be impossible) but to let it be known that review of these negative discussions and negative peer influence are part of the design. It is everyone's responsibility as close family members to bring these things out in a group so that the community remains positive and personal growth can be promoted.

Members and staff alike act as facilitators emphasizing people's personal responsibility for improving themselves and improving others. It is an unwritten rule in the TC that staff and members should not "do for" each other. They must encourage each other to "do for" themselves. Guidance, words of support, encouragement and even heavy confrontation are all part of this **facilitator role**. Again, this staff role differs dramatically from the "do for" roles of most staff members in most institutions where their job is to give pills to patients, to give services to patients, to supply food for patients, to clean patients' rooms, to take patients out for walks or recreation, etc. Members of the TC provide their own meals, clean their own rooms, create and plan their own recreation, activities and seminars, and provide for their own therapy and personal improvement.

Central to the TC is the concept of **experiential learning**. While didactic learning is present, learning from experience usually has the most lasting effect. Consistent with the normal process of growing up, the TC promotes a normal learning process whereby people can make mistakes but will learn from them. Trial and error failing and succeeding seems to promote lasting life style change. People are given a chance for real or legitimate success; a positive reinforcement which continually builds self-confidence.

There is a constant dialectical process ongoing in the TC between the individual needs and the group needs. The group and the community give the individuals the support, structure and self-respect that are needed to make it in the real world. During his process of inculcation of group values, however, individual preference and rebellion occur. Many TC staff members do not understand the need for this rebelliousness and so it is dealt with by hard confrontation and strong constraints to conform. Trained TC staff understand the need for people to express individuality as part of the growth process. Eventually some of the positive group norms and values are internalized, adding strength and confidence to the member. Rather than being extinguished, individual needs are channeled in a positive direction, i.e., that of preparing vocational, educational or career plans, understanding certain physical, medical or psychiatric needs that one person has but another person may not have, etc. Staff members know that the individual is the one who will make it in the real world, not the group. The individual must internalize group norms and values within the context of his/her own individuality.

The TC concept supports a **"no we-they dichotomy."** There is not room for "I'm better than you." Granted, some individuals may know more than others about some things, but everyone has his/her own knowledge to contribute and no one puts himself above the next person. Both staff and members work together on the same level in promoting the concepts of personal growth and the ideals of the community. There is some dichotomy here in that staff are paid and members are not, but the concept of a flat hierarchy is unique to a TC especially in comparison to a mental hospital.

Another concept that defines the TC is the concept of **"act as if."** In a mental institution or hospital, a person's attitudinal or behavioral comportment is accepted as part of his/her pathology or problem. In other words, that is why he/she is here. In the TC a morose attitude and negative behavior are not tolerated for any length of time. While despondence and depression may be natural and even a way of life for TC members, it is also contagious and can pass quickly through the entire community. If a member is sad, he/she is encouraged to act happy. If a member is angry, he/she is encourage to act serene. If a member is stubborn, he/she is encouraged to act more flexible. If a member is belligerent and refuses to acknowledge another point of view, he/she is encouraged to show understanding of other's ideas and values. An "act as if" attitude is encouraged 24 hours a day, not just during a group. While it may be hard to understand how this works, it is surprising that it works effectively and with less effort by members than might be imagined. With the concept of understanding, members quickly see another member's problems and notice that member "acting as if." It is easier then for that member to model his/her behavior after another member who really has something to be despondent over and does not let it affect his/her entire behavior and attitude.

This leads to the concept of role modeling. If members are not positive role models, the TC cannot work. The "act as if" supports the concept of the positive role model and positive modeling behavior has one of the strongest impacts on promoting lasting change and positive growth.

In every TC there must be a **system of beliefs** similar to societal norms or community values. These beliefs must be derived from the members and staff themselves and should not necessarily be imposed by program doctrine or a charismatic leader. In this way, the TC can be modified, evolving to meet changing norms and values of the larger society so that the TC microcosm is always in tune and better prepares members for their role in the larger society. There are no constraints on the specifics of the belief system. It must adhere to the TC code of ethics and bill of rights and fit the generic TC definition and concepts presented in the Therapeutic Community Training Manual.

Unlike mental hospitals, the TC tends to set higher expectations for its members, fostering more positive attitudes and achievement. Naturally these expectations must be based on reality, but TCs have found over the years that members can make tremendous strides in their own personal growth far beyond the expectations of traditional psychotherapy. In psychotherapy or psychiatry an individual's background plays a great role in future expectations for that person. In the TC, while the background material is important, present behavior and attitude is most important and high future expectations serve as motivators for greater achievement.

The Therapeutic Community Staff Development and Certification Process

Therapeutic Communities of America has codified the TC concept by defining it and by establishing basic knowledge or competence areas for the purpose of training and certification. The board of Therapeutic Communities of America has established the Certification Manual to define basic minimum criteria of competency in the field of TC counseling. The Therapeutic Communities of America certification process recognizes a staff member's competency as defined in this manual and the TCA board of directors approves three years certification for those staff members who have achieved the minimum skill or competence level.

The process of certification is a peer review process including a knowledge section, a written documentation section and a face-to-face interview section. There are three levels of review of the submitted certification package and no staff member of any agency can sign off initially on a certification package without having undergone the TCA certification evaluator's training. When an individual completes the certification requirements and is approved by the Certification Board of Directors, he/she receives Level 1 certification for a duration of three years. After this time period, this individual may renew his/her certification for another three years as long as his/her counseling status remains the same and the recertification fee is submitted. If that individual wants to advance his/her certification level, he/she must show evidence of having completed a certain number of hours of training, particularly in the areas relating to the evaluation of his/her Level 1 certification manual. In the three year period, the individual must accumulate a minimum of 60 contact hours of training relating to the TC in order to be approved for the Level 2 certification. Level 3 certification works in similar fashion. In addition to the Certification Manual's use as a training and staff development tool, TCA has recorded a 35-minute training tape.

Since 1981 when all the certification materials became available, programs in the United States and Canada have been using both the manual and the tape for the purposes of staff certification and training. In recent years these materials have been used by TCs worldwide in countries such as New Zealand, Brasil, Ireland, England, Italy, Holland and Germany as staff development and training tools.

Notes

1. For more information regarding the Therapeutic Community certification and staff development program, write to "TCC, P.O. Box 1806, Newark, NJ 07101," or call (201) 623-0600, extension 139.

CHAPTER 6

STRUCTURE, VARIATIONS, AND CONTEXT: A SOCIOLOGICAL VIEW OF THE THERAPEUTIC COMMUNITY

BARRY SUGARMAN

INTRODUCTION

THE THERAPEUTIC community (TC) phenomenon has been around a considerable time, since the late 1940s in its democratic version and since the late 1960s in its hierarchical (Concept House) version. The purpose of this article will be (1) to analyze the structure of the TC, examining features common to both versions as well as those that differentiate them and (2) to examine some of the contextual factors which account for differences in the growth of the TC movement in its different branches.

To understand the TC in the larger social context, the significance of differences between the two branches of the TC movement and their different historical development, as well as the dynamics of interaction between TC and the larger professional, social, and political environment, it is necessary to take a broad sociological view of the TC phenomenon.

In short, this article offers a sociological view of the TC with two goals. One is to define more adequately the structural elements for the benefit of those whose job it is to make the TC work as well as possible. The second goal is to get some perspective on the significance of the TC in the wider context of larger society.

Structure and Variations

This section examines the social structure of the TC to define the areas of difference between the democratic and hierarchical versions in relation to the common characteristics shared by both versions. J.K.W. Morrice noted in 1979 that the four "fundamental themes" stated by Rapoport in 1960 are still "worthy of general acceptance" (p. 40): democratization, permissiveness, reality confrontation and communalism. Morrice does not say so, but evidently he is writing on behalf of the democratic TC. To what extent are his four themes valid for the hierarchical (Concept) TC? On the face of it, two out of four apply (reality confrontation and commonalism) while two seem more questionable (democratization and permissiveness). For example, Rapoport defines democratization to mean the inclusion of clients in the treatment of other clients — both to help implement it and to help in making decisions about it. The hierarchical TC would rate "yes" on implementing but generally "no" on decision-making — except in the case of senior clients.

I believe a more detailed list of structural characteristics will help identify differences and commonalities. This section presents fifteen components and reviews how each applies to the two types of TC.

1. Behavioral Limits and Sanctions

All models of the TC involve a set of explicit behavior norms which members support and a set of contingent sanctions, positive and negative. Sanctions may range from informal disapproval to a formal vote of censure or a verbal haircut, from loss of privileges to demotion in status or even expulsion. Within this broad statement, though, there are wide differences between TCs of the democratic and hierarchical models. The hierarchical programs have extensive and demanding limits, strictly enforced, on the grounds that addicts need to learn self-control, and to experience the security of a firm framework of order. It is further maintained that, given extreme manipulativeness, they will undermine any organization that is not very tightly regulated. The democratic programs maintain that such behavior changes are temporary and worthless, that such demands alienate clients and drive them away from treatment, and that they are philosophically repugnant. They attempt to develop norms by consensus through democratic group process, which should result in more durable learning. While good results have been obtained in democratic TCs for many kinds of clients, evidence is lacking to support the success of this approach with addicts. There are reports of failure (Kooyman).

2. Positive Peer Pressure

Within the framework of group norms and sanctions outlined in the previous section, the TC goes further by mobilizing the forces of peer social pressure in their support. Not leaving matters just to the spontaneous group dynamics, all TCs reward residents who work to support the norms of the TC. They receive at least the approval and recognition of staff, as well as privileges and status advancement. Hierarchical TCs go farthest in the engineering of positive peer pressure by demanding that residents monitor the conduct of peers and confront them about failings — both one-to-one and in group settings. They are also required to participate in the organized group pressuring of deviants in haircuts, general meetings of certain individuals, etc.

These methods would be effective in any group, but especially with a group of addicts because they tend to be conformists. They lack the strong ego necessary to resist group pressure and indoctrination. Of course, their manipulativeness always threatens the group but in the well-organized hierarchical TC much of these characteristics are channelled into "playing the system" and to help maintain the positive peer pressure on each other (Sugarman).

Behavioral limits and sanctions plus **positive peer pressure** engender a short-term process of behavior modification. Even though this changed behavior is dependent upon the external controls of the social setting, still it has a real significance. Firstly, it creates and sustains the therapeutic milieu which is necessary for all further levels of learning and personal growth. Secondly, it signals to the resident a message which is the key to further growth. The message is: you **can** change in ways you would not have thought possible (Sugarman; Casriel).

3. Helping Each Other

- Helping another is the best way to help oneself.
- The help of a peer, a recent fellow-sufferer, is worth more than the help of an academically trained professional who lacks the common experience.

These twin precepts capture the essense of the mutual help principle which is fundamental to all TC models and, indeed to the whole movement of mutual help groups following the example of Alcoholics Anonymous (q.v.) (Lieberman & Borman). Helping each other includes both helping peers to struggle with their personal difficulties and helping them to perform their new roles in the TC. The latter is, in effect, a powerful form of informal, on-the-job training.

Through the mutual help process the following learning can occur, expressed in parallel statements from the perspective of helper and help-ee respectively, of course, each person plays both roles at different times — that is the whole point.

The **helper** learns	The **helpee** learns
— To help another person and hence to see that one can be important in the life of another person.	— Someone can understand me.
	— Someone cares enough to do so.
	— Help is available for the asking.
— To strengthen one's own commitment to change.	— In the TC certain kinds of help/ pressure/confrontation will be given whether we want them or
— To feel pride in one's progress so far.	not.

4. Confrontation

Helping within the Therapeutic Community takes many forms, many of them common to other mutual help organizations. Confrontation is a distinctive form of peer helping crucial to the TC. All groups of any kind — depend on social feedback, meaning communication back to a member on how his/her prior actions are perceived or how they impact on oneself (the source of the feedback). Confrontation **a la** TC involves delivering feedback which is needed but not welcomed by the recipient and hence is very difficult for the donor. Confrontation is the powerful antiseptic which TC residents use to clean the many wounds and sores on themselves and on others, some still open, others closed up but infected beneath. It is painful even though essential for recovery. There are intriguing historical precedents in utopian communities such as the Oneida (Nordhof). The courage to take the medicine of self-confrontation and to accept the helping confrontations of others, turning them into true self-confrontations, is the ultimate factor in determining the success of the Therapeutic Community experience.

What articulates part of this notion is more recent psychological thinking about the essential role of a sense of efficacy and competence in healthy individual development (Kent and Rolf). It is this sense which is cultivated through constructive activity and achievement regardless of the specific content — whether it be helping parents in a family-operated farm or business, repairing old cars, or studying for an exam and passing.

Note that the activity may be solitary or done as part of a group. In either case the recognition of others is an important part of the reinforcement or reward. The social factor involved in **group** activities adds an important dimension to the growth value of the experience because it is affirming the competence of the individual as a **social** person. In the TC, constructive activity is promoted mainly as a group experience.

Through constructive activity and achievement, pride and a sense of self-worth develops, based on the recognition of competence by self and others. Good work habits are also developed through this learning process.

5. Living in a Self-Sufficient Group

Because the TC is a **self-sufficient** group, this endows any work for the group with a further important quality. Just as the crew of a small boat on the open sea, or a band of explorers in the wilderness, depends for their very lives on each person performing his/her responsibilities adequately, so too do members of the TC depend upon each one carrying out assigned responsbilities.

The self-sufficient group is a particularly important setting for learning the nature of social responsibility and the interdependence of individual interests. Ideally, the ordinary family and the ordinary peer groups a child experiences in growing up convey this kind of learning; in practice, the lesson is often missed either due to social disorganization or to the misguided efforts of over-indulgent parents to protect their children from normal expectations that they fulfill their responsibilities. In the deliberately isolated social structure of the TC, the individual has to face the fact that his/her neglect of responsibilities threatens the welfare of others and hence leads to sanctions from them, including confrontation. Whereas in the complex mass society, the parasite can hide from the consequences of ignoring the needs of others, this is made impossible in the TC.

The degree to which self-sufficiency is structured into the TC varies. All set a boundary around their life-space and encapsulate it (see item 10). Some go farther than others in the degree to which the subsistence of the group depends directly on the efforts of residents. Thus some TCs grow their own food with resident labor or solicit contributions with resident help. Internally, preparing meals for the group and repainting or renovating the building represents the same experience. To the degree that TCs hire paid staff to perform these functions, they diminish an important learning opportunity. Some earlier (pre-TC) programs were based entirely on this principle of moral education through living in a self-sufficient community, such as the Junior Republics and the socialist youth projects associated with Makarenko (Bazeley; Mann and Wingard; Makerenko).

6. Open System Communication

This aspect is considered in two parts: (1) sharing of information and (2) sharing of decision-making authority. The first part (sharing of information) is quite widely agreed to be an important requirement of the TC, even between proponents of the hierarchical and democratic models. This applies most strongly to information about the residents' behavior and their problems, which is shared with amazing thoroughness. Privacy is a negative value in the TC. Mutual help requires this shared knowledge, though, and the effective monitoring of behavior for prevention of deviance requires it too. In administrative areas the hierarchical TCs share information less freely than democratic ones. The latter must share this very fully because they allow residents the right to be involved in decision-making. In hierarchical TCs, administrative (non-clinical) information is often disclosed on a limited (need-to-know) basis or is announced to the whole body, often at the last moment. Sharing of information is not a fully consensual area between TCs of the two basic types, but more so than the area of decision-making authority, where we find a major disagreement.

The hierarchical model officially reserves decision-making to those who hold positions in the authority structure. Informally or in staff meetings, a director will often consult with those on one or even two levels below him/her but is not required to do so. Rarely indeed will there ever be an open meeting with residents for discussion of an issue of clinical or administrative policy. Never would an important decision be put to a vote of residents. By contrast the democratic model uses the daily community meeting of staff and residents as an open forum for discussion and the staff meetings as an open deliberative body operating on major issues by consensus (Jones). There is much use of two-way communication in the democratic model.

Later it will be suggested that at different phases of treatment the most appropriate patterns for involving residents (including junior staff) in decision-making may vary. This could also be a basis for achieving more consensus between the two schools of thought which still divide on the general issue of decision-making authority in the TC.

7. Limited Communication Outside Therapeutic Community

The TC operates as a small world unto itself, sheltered from contact with the outside world in many ways. The purpose of this is to intensify the group dynamics and all the learning processes engendered here. It is also to prevent interference or contamination from the outside, for example to control opportunities to acquire contraband, to plan escapes, or to talk with those who might be "negative" influences.

While tight boundaries seem necessary in the early phase of residence, when prolonged this isolation tends to create the typical effects of institutionalization which require costly efforts to reverse them when preparing the resident for reentry.

8. Use of Pressure to Recruit and Hold Clients

This issue, like the previous one, represents disagreement between the two TC traditions or models. The hierarchical model emphasizes the self-destructiveness, impulsiveness, and irresponsibility of the addict and hence the impossibility of helping him without some use of external pressure initially. This is often in the form of a suspended jail sentence liable to be imposed in the event of leaving the TC without permission or failing to cooperate. Even this degree of pressure is far from sure to hold the addict in treatment. If he/she does stay, the motivation must change from external pressure to intrinsic value. The democratic model opposes this approach on grounds of civil liberties.

9. Counseling

Informal counseling is included above under "helping others." More formal counseling also has a significant role in the TC. This may be done by academically trained persons (either staff or as part-time consultants) or by indigenous staff.

Family counseling is an area of special interest since it goes beyond the simple model of the TC as an enclosed social group. The skills required for family counseling are not the same as those needed for the counseling of residents in-house. Aftercare counseling also requires a different set of skills (Bratter, 1981).

When successful, counseling helps the recipient to achieve clearer **insight** into self, feelings, motives, and conflicts. It helps him/her to clarify goals and values, and to make appropriate plans to achieve them. It helps to identify and to resolve or to accept contradictions in one's life. These processes are less important in the early stages of treatment but become extremely important in the middle and later stages.

10. Education and Formal Skill Training

A resident with serious educational deficits may begin work on reme-
diation usually after initial adjustment to the TC setting. Rather than
detracting from his basic personal growth — as feared by some early
Concept House Directors — a good basic education program usually
enhances personal growth in the TC.

Analogous to the above it is possible and desirable for TCs to intro-
duce other kinds of formal skill training to meet specific deficits of residents in non-academic areas. Because many kinds of skill learning have
traditionally been embedded in the TC experience, such as assertive-
ness, supervisory skills, counseling skills, and various job-related skills
for in-house jobs, two important assumptions have easily been made.
One is that this informal learning covers **all** significant non-academic
skills by residents and the other is that this is an adequate means of
learning those areas so covered. Both assumptions are open to question.

11. Supervised Outside Contact

Given the principle of limited communication outside the TC, this
still does not necessitate total isolation. Outside contacts, appropriately
supervised, can be quite well controlled and therapeutic in outcome,
whether they occur by visitors coming to the TC or by TC residents going outside.

12. Organized Recreation

Addicts have typically never learned to use leisure time without
drugs or to have fun in drug-free ways. The same is probably true of
other TC client groups. Before they are ready to leave the TC, therefore, something (e.g. seminars, organized activities) needs to be provided in this area. A regular place within the TC schedule must be
assigned to help residents develop leisure interests, and specific staff
given this responsibility. Given a recognition of these objectives, all staff
members should be encouraged to contribute, for example, by sending
residents outside for ten minutes to watch the sunset.

13. Preaching and Public Confession

Enormous amounts of time and energy in the TC are spent in preaching and in being preached at. All of this effort probably does more good
for the preachers than it does for the recipients. A special kind of preaching is that done by the penitent, making public confession. Mowrer has
noted the special importance of this open confession and even Oscar

Wilde commented, "It is the confession, not the priest, that gives us absolution." The public confession, linked with the public commitment to personal change in specified ways, is a major feature of the TC.

Preaching includes both the exhortation of others to change and the articulation of the TC philosophy, beliefs, and values. This is important in an educational sense, helping residents to understand better a set of ideas which is extensive and subtle, even while many of the central ideas can be expressed very simple. Differences in emphasis are found among TCs in the balance they strike between two themes in their preaching. One theme is that of **hope** for a brighter personal future as the result of present struggles; the other theme is that of **fear** of returning to the old life and fear of disaster if the resident should give up the struggle to change. While hierarchical programs tend to make heavier use of fear psychology in their preaching, both themes are found in both types of programs.

For the preacher or confessor him/herself these activities tend to strengthen commitment to the values and goals expressed. The listeners may learn more about the group philosophy. Last but not least, these activities contribute to the peer pressure phenomenon.

14. Ritual Participation

Life in the TC involves various ritual activities, repeated events which always have a predictable form and sequence, in which residents are participants not merely observers. Such events include: Community meetings of the entire membership and staff with their opening and closing rituals, the initiation of new members, graduation, and public reprimands. These events become familiar and they give concrete meaning to the abstract concepts acquired through preaching. Their familiarity creates a sense of belonging and group cohesiveness.

15. Spirituality and the "Higher Power" Concept

Since the TC draws so much from the mutual help principle of Alcoholics Anonymous (AA) it is instructive to note an area of great difference — and one that I believe needs more attention. AA teaches recovering alcoholics to trust in a "higher power" who will fortify their efforts in the daily struggle to remain abstinent. TCs with very few exceptions, eliminate any reference to religion, duty, or any such "higher power." While it can be argued that the TC experience is so much more powerful than the AA experience that TC residents do not need such a "crutch," the experience of TC residents after treatment, while it is impressive, is not so close to 100 percent that we can afford to reject anything that might strengthen it. We must explore whether there is a hidden cost to including the "higher power" concept. To some thinkers it may seem to detract from the pure emphasis on self-determination; to others this is an exaggerated emphasis anyway (Alcoholics Anonymous; Wilson).

Table 1

STRUCTURAL COMPONENTS OF THE TC AS EMPHASIZED
IN THE HIERARCHICAL AND DEMOCRATIC VERSIONS
OF THE MODEL RESPECTIVELY

Components	Hierarchical Model	Democratic Model	Same "*" or Different "-"
1. Behavioral limits & sanctions	× ×	×	–
2. Positive peer pressure	× ×	×	–
3. Helping each other	× ×	× ×	*
4. Confrontation	× ×	× ×	*
5. Living in a self-sufficient group	×	×	*
6. Open) a) information sharing system) communic.)	×	× ×	–
b) shared decision-making	0	× ×	– –
7. Insulation from outside forces	×	×	*
8. Pressures used to recruit & hold clients	× ×	×	–
9. Counseling	× ×	× ×	*
10. Education & formal skill training	× ×	× ×	*
11. Supervised community contact	× ×	× ×	*
12. Organized recreation	?	?	*
13. Preaching & public confession	× ×	×	–
14. Ritual participation	× ×	× ×	*
15. Concept of a "higher power"	?	?	?

Table 1 summarizes the discussion of this section, listing the fifteen structural components and indicating for each of the two major TC variations (democratic and hierarchical) whether the component is usually found in

- an important role (× ×)
- a moderately important role (×)
- few examples of unimportance (0).

We have, then, a comparative structural profile of the two major types of TC.

The third column of Table 1 makes line by line comparisons, starting those when the two types match "*" and marking those where they do not match with "-." It does **not** make sense to treat this as a scale with equally weighted items and compute a score of "matches" minus "no-matches." Certainly these components are not all of equal weight but we have not determined how to weight them. All we can conclude in a quantitative form is that the two models match on nine components and disagree on five. One of the five is a two-part item which could be counted as two-making six "disagree."

Clearly, there are certain characteristics which are very important in both types and which differentiate both types of TC from other treatment methods.

These are:

- mutual help
- confrontation
- ritual participation

Other shared characteristics which are only moderately important to both are:

- living in a self-sufficient group
- insulation from outside forces

There are other shared characteristics which are important to the TC (both types) but which differentitate the TC from many non-TC methods. These are: counseling (formal), education and formal skill training, supervised; community contact, (maybe) organized recreation, and (maybe) "higher power."

We find structural differences between the two models of TC in five or six areas. Only one out of six is a plus-to-minus difference; all others are differences between **very** and **moderately** important. Features that are very important in the hierarchical model and less important in the democratic model are:

- behavioral limits and sanctions
- positive peer pressure
- pressure used to recruit and hold clients
- preaching and public confession.

Only one feature is very important in the democratic model and less important in the hierarchical model:

- information sharing

Finally there is one feature of utmost importance to the democratic model but not accepted in the hierarchical model:

- shared decision-making

In addition to this analysis of typological differences, our list of structural components can serve as a check-list for future TC architects to use. In designing future TCs it will surely be important to consider systematically each of the structural characteristics reviewed above. In future models there may be good grounds for "rebuilding" the inherited models and putting together some new model consisting of a different package of key structural components.

In an earlier paper (Sugarman, 1984) I have related these **two** types of TCs to **two phases** in the rehabilitation process, suggesting that the ideal TC, synthesizing the wisdom of both types, combines a relatively hierarchical structure in the early phases of the process and shifts to a more democratic structure in the later phases — especially reentry.

The TC in its Larger Social Context

The TC makes a radical break from traditional approaches to treatment, rehabilitation, counseling, education, social work, etc. It presents a strikingly different model of professional work, new ways of communicating and using feedback, new authority patterns, new definitions of responsibility, new visions of human growth and potential.

While the relentless trend of increasing specialization has affected all medial, social, and educational services, the TC has taken the diametrically opposite approach. The TC brings a wholistic approach that addresses the whole person — not just his different diseases or problems; it addresses that person in a micro-community that operates in a unified way. The internal milieu of the TC is carefully monitored and managed, as the major treatment resource. In a pluralistic society in which cohesive communities for most people are a long past memory (or myth), the TC functions as a cohesive, bounded, nurturing but demanding group, somewhat like an extended family or peer group living together.

This sociological uniqueness would make the TC an extremely important phenomenon, even if there were no evidence to show that it produced favorable outcomes for graduates. Since there is such evidence anyhow (see this volume) the TC becomes doubly important.

As a radically new approach in human services, the TC has experienced similar mixed responses to those experienced by many other significant social innovations — uncritical admiration in some quarters, ridicule and overt opposition in others, covert sabotage, surface adoption and dilution of the real essence.

A "social" innovation is one which affects the social balance, the relationships of status, power, and material gain between people and groups. Because the TC aims **directly** at those relationships one could hardly expect it to have an easy time. The first point to make, then, is that the mere fact that it survived at all is remarkable. That must be considered an indication of two things: effective leadership in the early years and the fact that the earliest TCs could be seen as the **only** possible answer to a critical need that was causing great concern to some people with significant power.

The TC phenomenon would probably not have happened without some remarkable leaders (Maxwell Jones, Charles Dederich, David Deitch, and others) but none of the pioneer TCs arose from clear, preconceived models in the heads of their founders — let alone explicit plans or proposals. In the early years, both in Britain at the end of World War II (Jones, 1984) and in California in the early 1960s (Yablonsky), creative leaders were responding to unusual crisis situations in the ways that their backgrounds and personalities predisposed them.

Jones, the British psychiatrist working within the government-supported medical system and Dederich, the American unemployed ex-salesman and recently recovering alcoholic operating completely on his own meager resources, both shared a strong antipathy to traditional authority patterns in medicine and human services plus a faith in the power of all kinds of people to help one another.

Social conditions were desperate when the early TC, deviant form that it was, made its first appearance — else it would not have been tolerated. In 1945 the British military needed to resettle over a thousand ex-POWS with severe mental disturbance (Jones, 1984). All facilities, were already grossly over-extended even before this on-slaught. Jones's unorthodox way of extending his slender resources through the TC approach was tolerated when it likely would have been forbidden in more normal times. In 1957 Long Beach, California alcoholics and addicts were desperate for help: Dederich's strange set-up was available and seemed to work (Casriel, Yablonsky). Meanwhile across the USA many judges, probation administrators, and other public officials — not to mention the general public — were also desperate to find a treatment for burgeoning narcotic addiction, and the apparently related crime wave. All traditional methods had patently failed.

So desperate was the criminal justice establishment in 1962 that a team set out from New York City, financed by NIMH, to cross the country investigating any approach to the treatment of narcotic addiction that offered any promise whatsoever (Bassin). The inclusion of Synanon on their itinerary was quite fortuitous but historically momentous. Shelly and Bassin, team leaders from the Probation Department of Brooklyn Supreme Court quickly wrote a grant proposal to NIMH for funding of a "half way house" for indicted addicts to be run along Synanon lives. They were quickly funded. After a couple of mistakes in staffing the directors position, Daytop Lodge was successfully established under the leadership of David Deitch, who had learned his job at Synanon.

Soon thereafter the Phoenix House program also began in New York City, another attempt to domesticate the Synanon magic. The first point of difference from Synanon, shared by both Daytop and Phoenix, was the contractual funding relationship with government agencies. Synanon refused to accept any "strings" attached to public funding and, therefore, never received any. If depended on its own private fundraising, in keeping with its evential posture as an alternative society rather than a mere rehabilitation program.

Having given birth to a new generation and a new type of TC, Synanon continued its own course. Dederich came to place more and more emphasis on Synanon's mission as an alternative (utopian) society — not a mere rehabilitation program, treating casualties so they might be sent back into the battlefield. Because of the personal pathologies of Dederich and the structural problem that there was no system of checks and balances in Synanon to rein him in. Synanon for a time acquired a reputation for interval despotism and for vicious attacks on external critics (Deitch and Sweben). Since Dederich's death, leadership has passed to his two children. Though little information has come out of Synanon in recent years regarding changes in policy, there are some indications of more moderation.

Our concern here is, however, more with the new branch of the TC movement. Having begun as a satellite program of the Brooklyn Supreme Court Probation Department, Daytop Village soon found this relationship to be a problem. Deitch wanted more freedom as TC leader than Shelly, Chief Probation Officer and project administrator, would or could allow. The solution to this problem was, with the agreement of NIMH, to create a private, non-profit corporation, "Daytop Village," with its own board of directors. This board, not Shelly, would be accountable to NIMH and other interested parties. They would take the heat in case of community outrage, law suit, etc. They permitted Deitch to admit females as well as males into the program, where Shelly had refused, and gave him other freedom — until the "Big Split" between director and board in 1968 (Bassi; Sugarman, 1974).

Daytop, Phoenix and many other Concept House TCs thrived between about 1965 and 1975. In 1977 Bassin estimated there were some 2,000 in the USA. In 1982 Sherry Holland found records at NIDA on over 1,000 residential drug-free programs. There are now third and fourth generations of TCs. The vast majority operate as free-standing agencies, with their own incorporation.

This appears to be a major and significant difference from the democratic TCs, often operating within a mental health host organization, having a pre-existing mission and power structure, which keeps the TC in a weak position.

In the drug addiction field in the USA the hierarchical TC is recognized a one of only two or three major treatment modalities, the others being methadone and the traditional medical approach. In this field, TCs moved into a power vacuum and established new, independent beachheads, taking over territory not already held by the medical world. In the field of mental health in the USA the status of the TC is quite inferior. Intellectually it is fairly widely known but either it is considered heterodox and threatening or, less often, it is superfically embraced in a half-hearted manner. In the latter case, the TC model is grossly abused by applying the name to any hospital unit where a community meeting is conducted in any shape or form.

During the years when TCs were being established and were flourishing as independent drug addiction treatment programs, the field of mental health was de-emphasizing in-patient programs in favor of "deinstitutionalization." Since the TC concept has, for much of its history been associated mainly with residential and in-patient settings, deinstitutionalization has weakened its influence in the mental health world.

The differential development of the two branches of the TC movement is a result of the different affiliations they each made with other social institutions. The Concept TCs, serving drug addicts in the USA, affiliated themselves primarily with the so-called criminal justice systems for recruitment of clients, while their funding usually came from grants of public funds. The mental hospital TCs affiliated with the health care system and typically operated in hospitals or under their control. Funding depended on whether the host hospital was publically funded or financed by fees from patients and insurance companies. In either case, the power structure of the health care system (including the medical establishement and the other conservative elements of the community) has played an important role in thwarting the growth of TCs, more often by forcing them to lapse into more traditional practices, rather than by closing down their beds. Whiteley's survey of British TCs in the mental health even confirms the low standing of TCs in this field (Hinshelwood and Manning, ch. 2)

The Concept TCs have most often been independent agencies with a board of directors commited to the TC approach. When they have faced irresistable pressure they have complied in some areas, such as installing better financial controls, keeping better clinical records, formal treatment planning, and staff credentialling. These pressures may be powerful, reinforced as they can be by the power of the purse. However, these are pressures on an independent agency. A TC that is not separately incorporated, such as one operating with a traditional hospital or prison, is open to even more pressures. For example, administrators of the host institution with authority over centralized services needed by the TC may refuse to cooperate and undermine the TC's control of its own setting; the physicians' grapevine may spread negative impressions, discouraging staff from working there and preventing referral of patients, and insurance companies may refuse to pay for treatment provided in non-traditional ways.

There is much more to be learned about the dynamic interplay between the TC and its larger social context. We have said nothing about the situation in European nations where national health care systems and more centralized social welfare systems constitute an environment very different from that of the USA. Comparative studies are warranted. Where Jones (1976) has advocated the use of open system concepts for understanding the dynamics of the TC, we have here taken an open system model as our conceptual framework for analyzing the interplay between the TC and its context.

Conclusion

This discussion has taken a sociological view of the TC, its structure and relationship to the larger social context. Looking at the distinctive structure of the TC, we first presented a list of eighteen structural components which we used to analyze differences between the democratic and hierarchical models and to establish the larger number of common components. This list of eighteen components may be used both for analysing existing TCs and for designing future ones.

Looking, secondly, at the relationship between the TC and its larger social context, we have attempted to understand how the TC, as a radical innovation, could have gained initial acceptance (or toleration) of its pilot projects; how the different branches of its TC movement affiliated with different institutions in the larger society, and how those affiliations affected the growth or restriction of the TC movement in its different branches. In particular we tried to learn something from the contrast between the success of TCs in the US drug addiction field and the lesser acceptance and growth of TCs in the US mental health field. Further research on the role of the TC model in adult and youth corrections is needed.

The TC can be seen as a major episode in the development of mental hospitals and revolution in the field of treatment for addiction. More broadly it can be seen as a major innovation in the human services, with applications in many fields. Maxwell Jones has emphasized the central importance of "social learning" in the TC, leading to the thought that "learning community" might be a more generic and relevant title. This term is already in use, designating an alternative model of formal education. Generically "Learning Community" might help to clarify the applicability of TC principles to personal growth and learning in many settings, without the clinical overtones of "therapeutic" (see Sugarman, 1974).

The significance of the TC lies in its power to harness the power of group dynamics to enhance the process of treatment or rehabilitation; in demystifying that process; in empowering both clients and all levels of staff; and in creating a context for wholistic caring and healing, where the client is treated as an individual person — not as a bundle of symptoms and problems.

In assessing the importance of the TC we must include its significance for its actual clients, for its intended clients, for the wider community which in effect sponsors it, and for the staff who work there. For a society which functions in a highly specialized, competitive, pluralistic fragmented, and materialistic way, yet which still cherishes the values of community and wholistic caring the TC offers an important oasis of these, older values.

"The Therapeutic Community is not a place, or just another tool of rehabilitation. It is a philosophy."

> *Dr. Theodore B. R. Abas, Vice-President,*
> *DARE Foundation, Inc. at 6th World Conference*
> *of Therapeutic Communities*

Part II

RESEARCH AND EVALUATION: OUTCOMES AND PROCESS

CHAPTER 7

THERAPEUTIC COMMUNITY RESEARCH: OVERVIEW AND IMPLICATIONS

GEORGE DE LEON, PH.D.

RECENT YEARS have witnessed a burdgeoning of research and evaluation in drug treatment. Studies mainly involve long term "traditional" TCs, although other varieties have been studied. The emphasis of this work has been on treatment outcome, with fewer investigations of retention and treatment process. This paper provides an overview of the main findings and conclusions from this research and outlines some implications for treatment, theory and further research.*

TREATMENT OUTCOME

The effectiveness of therapeutic communities has been evaluated primarily through follow-up studies. Many of these have been executed by investigative teams engaged in large scale modality comparisons that include therapeutic communities. Others have been conducted on and by individual TCs. Most studies utilized self report which was considered reliable, although several contain corroborating information from outside agencies.

Social Adjustment: All of the studies revealed that immediate and long-term outcome status of the clients followed are significantly improved over pre-treatment status. Drug use and criminality declined

---

*The literature isn't exhaustively surveyed, nor is it critically reviewed. Although attention was placed on recent research, the bibliography includes references that extend back to 1969. With few exceptions, the papers cited in the text are those reported after 1977. Much of the material in this review is drawn from De Leon, 1984b.

while measures of prosocial behavior (employment and/or school in-volvement) increased (Barr & Antes, 1981; Brook & Whitehead, 1980; De Leon, 1984a; De Leon et al., 1972, 1979; Holland, 1978; Pompi et al., 1979; Wilson & Mandelbrote, 1978, Simpson & Sells, 1982).

A few studies have utilized a composite index of successful outcome, combining measures of criminal activity, drug use and employment. In these, maximally of moderately favorable outcome occurred in approxi-mately half the clients followed (De Leon, 1984a; Simpson & Sells, 1982).

Psychological Adjustment: Although a primary goal of therapeutic communities is psychological adjustment, this domain appears in few outcomes studies (Brook & Whitehead, 1980; De Leon, 1984a; De Leon & Jainchill, 1981-82; Kennard & Wilson, 1979). In these, psychological scores or profiles significantly improved at follow-up. Phoenix House studies have also demonstrated a direct correlation between social ad-justment (success rates) and psychological adjustments at two-year follow-up (De Leon, 1984a; De Leon & Jainchill, 1981-82).

Time in Program: Studies which examined differences between clients who complete (graduates) and drop out of treatment indicated that the graduates were significantly better than dropouts on all measures of outcome. The investigations that analyzed time in program (TIP) reported a positive relationship between favorable outcome and length of stay in treatment among dropouts (see Figure 1) (Barr & Antes, 1981; Coombs, 1981; De Leon, 1984a; Holland, 1983; Simpson & Sells, 1982; Wilson & Mandelbrote, 1978).

Who are the Successes?: Research has yet to delineate a client pro-file that predicts successful outcome. Age, race and other demographic factors do not relate to outcome in TCs. In Phoenix House research, fe-males do yield significantly better psychological adjustment than males at follow-up (De Leon & Jainchill, 1981-82). However, this difference in psychological outcome by sex remains to be replicated in other pro-grams.

Several background correlates of positive outcomes on drug use, criminality or employment have been identified, e.g., lower lifetime criminality, higher pretreatment educational level, opioid as a primary drug (De Leon, 1983a; Simpson & Sells, 1982). Though significant, these associations were small when compared with the effects of time in program; nor are they strong predictors of successful status measured with a composite index.

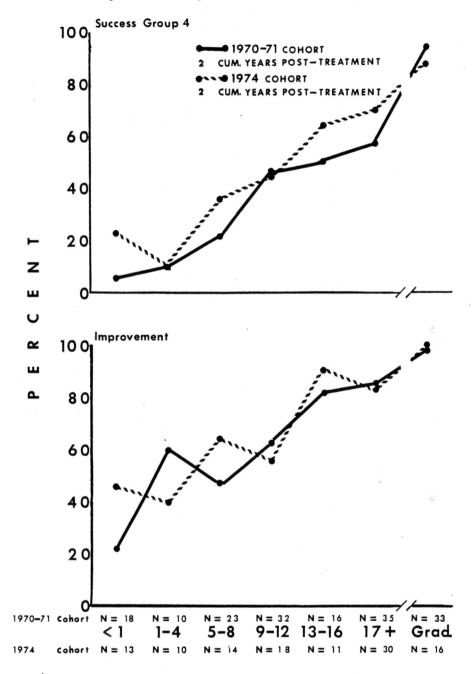

Figure 1. Success and improvement rates.

RETENTION

Time in program is the most consistent predictor of successful out-come. This finding stresses the importance of understanding retention as a phenomenon in its own right. Thus far, however, research has not yielded clear answers to three main retention questions: What are the retention rates? Who are the dropouts? And, why do clients leave or re-main in treatment?

No client profile has emerged which predicts length of stay in treat-ment. Research reveals only sporadic and weak correlates of dropout in-volving demographic, primary drug, background characteristics, pre-treatment status and psychological adjustment. Generally, however, social background (lifetime) characteristics have not predicted long-term retention, with the exception of less severe criminality.

Client status in the months prior to treatment is more closely related to retention. For example, those under legal pressure or whose health or lifestyle appears to have worsened, reveal somewhat longer durations of stay in TCs (Condelli, 1983; De Leon, 1983a; Holland, 1982).

Simiarly, psychological profiles on entry into treatment fail to predict overall retention in treatment, although psychological factors still ap-pear to be important. For example, several investigations indicate that early dropouts reveal higher levels of psychological dysfunction measured with standard paper and pencil instruments (De Leon et al., 1973; Sacks & Levy, 1979; Wexler & De Leon, 1977; Zuckerman et al., 1975). Some studies suggest that clients who showed less defensiveness and less denial of problems remain longer in treatment (De Leon, 1983a; Washburn, 1979).

One impressive finding obtained in a recent investigation involving a consortium of therapeutic communities revealed a striking relationship between psychological change during treatment and overall retention. Individuals who psychologically improved within the first several months after admission showed a significantly greater likelihood of con-tinuing their stay in treatment (De Leon, 1980a). This finding has obvi-ous implications for clarifying the relationship between client progress and retention.

Retention rates in therapeutic communities have received some at-tention in the literature (Brook & Whitehead, 1980; De Leon & Sch-wartz, 1984; Glaser, 1974; Sansone, 1980). The pattern of retention in long- term therapeutic communities is orderly and predictable. Dropout is highest within the first 15 days of admission and declines sharply thereafter so that the likelihood of dropout decreases with length of stay itself.

Why clients drop out of treatment is a question that has not been adequately investigated, although hypotheses concerning dropout have been offered mainly from clinical impressions (Baekland & Lundwall, 1975; De Leon, 1984b; De Leon & Rosenthal, 1979; Heit & Pompi, 1977; Sansone, 1980). In Phoenix House follow-up studies, analyses of clients' retrospective reasons for dropout distributed equally between those relating to program problems (e.g., conflict with staff, views of treatment) and those that were more personal (e.g., wanted to continue using drugs, wanted to work). Program versus personal reasons differed by length of stay, with significantly fewer personal reasons associated with retention over 12 months in treatment (De Leon, 1984c).

Studies involving other therapeutic communities highlight the importance of the client's perception of self, the environment and circumstance in relation to dropout. For example, clients who enter treatment under legal or family pressure remained longer only if they perceive those pressures as negative (Condelli, 1983).

TREATMENT PROCESS

Treatment process has been the least investigated problem in drug abuse treatment research. Ironically, the first process studies in TCs appeared more than a decade ago but their importance receded in favor of the need to establish firm information concerning treatment effectiveness. The relatively few process studies in the literature may be classified into three categories: studies of treatment change, direct investigations of treatment elements and client attribution of treatment influences.

Psychological Change: Studies have examined clients' psychological change during stay in programs without assessment of treatment components. They are reviewed as process studies since many of the psychological scores measuring change reflected program goals, e.g., attitudes, ego strength, emotional control, responsibility, self esteem, etc. Together with behavioral changes in drug use and anti-social behavior, these psychological changes during residency have strengthened inferences concerning the specific influences of treatment elements.

The studies employed standardized psychological instruments but vary with respect to design, number of variables measured and the number of observations during treatment (Biase, 1981; Brook & Whitehead, 1980; De Leon, 1974, 1976, 1980a; De Leon, et al., 1971, 1973; Kennard & Wilson, 1979; Sacks & Levy, 1979; Zuckerman et al., 1975). However, results are quite uniform in showing: (a) the profiles or pattern of psychological scores is similar across programs and even even cultures. For example, prominent are the signs of character disorder, personality inadequacy, mood disorder, poor self esteem and dull-normal intellectual level; (b) overall psychological status improves significantly during treatment across most measures but generally does not attain normative or healthy levels. Larger improvements occur in self esteem, ego strength, socialization and depression. Relatively smaller changes occur in the more enduring personality features, e.g., the character disorder elements. Thus, drug abusers in the TC are psychologically similar and show significant improvement in most psychological domains, although long standing character traits are more resistant to change; (c) psychological improvement post treatment generally exceed the gains made during treatment.

Studies completed at Phoenix House specifically correlated behavioral indices of drug use and crime (success status) with psychological improvement during treatment and at follow-up. Clients with an unfavorable success index at follow-up showed little psychological change during treatment or at follow-up. In contrast, clients who obtained a favorable success index had revealed significant psychological improvement during treatment and continued psychological gains at follow-up. This important finding offers indirect but positive evidence for the influence of treatment factors in the change process.

Treatment Elements: Some studies have addressed the relationship between specific treatment elements and client change during residential treatment. For example, results show significant reductions in self rated emotionality (depression, hostility, anxiety) and in physiological "upset" (systolic blood pressure) immediately following participation in encounter therapy sessions when compared with baseline measures (Biase & De Leon, 1969; De Leon & Biase, 1975).

Research in progress at Daytop Village therapeutic community has experimentally evaluated the effects of a specific educational intervention (college credit courses) upon clients in a therapeutic community. Findings support TC assumptions concerning treatment process and role changes. The students revealed significantly enhanced self esteem over that expected from treatment effects alone in the TC (Biase, 1981).

Treatment process has been indirectly examined in studies of client perception of the therapeutic community environment (Bell, 1983; De Leon, et al., 1980). Although preliminary, the results obtained across several programs are stable and orderly. All TC programs revealed a characteristic environmental profile that differed from hospitals and jails; and client perceptions of the environment were consistent with expectation concerning treatment change and length of stay. These findings support assumptions that traditional TCs are similar in philosophy, structure and practices.

Attribution: These studies have investigated client perceptions of their experiences in TCs. Generally, on measures of satisfaction, clients report a favorable experience in the therapeutic community and would recommend their particular residential program to others (De Leon, 1984c; Simpson & Lloyd, 1979; Winick, 1980). For example, successful follow-up status and length of stay in treatment significantly related to satisfaction with treatment, the relevance of specific program components to follow-up status and client weighting of the relative importance of treatment and non-treatment influences upon their lifestyles since leaving treatment (De Leon, 1984c). Although clear, these findings must be cautiously interpreted, given their retrospective nature. Possible halo effects, or dissonance factors might have influenced client perception of treatment experience and their own follow-up status. Nevertheless, the results firmly support hypotheses concerning the relationships between treatment experience, treatment elements and outcome status.

SUMMARY

There are several conclusions from the review of the literature. **First,** a substantial number of admissions to TCs reveal favorable or improved behavioral and psychological status at follow-up. Notably, the percentage of positive outcomes increases directly with time spent in treatment. However, research has yet to describe a client profile that predicts successful outcome; and only a few variables are consistent predictors of outcome other than length of stay. **Second,** dropout is the rule across TCs (and other drug treatment modalities) and the temporal pattern of dropout is predictable; most admissions leave treatment before maximally benefical effects are rendered. However, relatively little is known about who drops out or remains in TCs. Typical client profiles in relation to retention have not been delineated and there are no variables that are consistent or large predictors of dropout. Research has not clarified the reasons from dropout, although studies point to the importance of the client's perception of the treatment environment and of their problems in influencing retention. **Third**, there is relatively little research on treatment process in TCs. The findings obtained support inferences concerning the process of change but the process itself remains to be investigated.

SOME IMPLICATIONS FOR RESEARCH AND TREATMENT

Perspective on Treatment Effectiveness: TCs are effective when evaluated in terms of their principle aim of modifying both social and psychological adjustment. However, this conclusion remains tentative in light of familiar methodological considerations, the most serious of which is the lack of control groups. The follow-up samples studied may be self selected to seek, remain in and benefit from the TCs or, perhaps to improve without any treatment. Thus far, however, solutions to these selection problems have eluded research strategies. There are ethical problems in withholding treatment; and assembling matched control or comparative treatment groups though random assignment has not been feasible.

The methodological difficulties stress the need for a revised perspective on the interpretation of treatment outcome research which would reflect the multivariate complexity of individual change. One such perspective has been outlined for therapeutic communities in other writing (De Leon, 1980b, 1984a; De Leon, et al., 1982). Briefly, successful outcome emerges from an interaction of client treatment and non-treatment influence. The specific impact of the treatment experience is most apparent during and immediately following residency; thereafter, though less recognizable treatment effects may integrate with (or perhaps alter) the contribution of later experiences in maintaining successful status.

This perspective emphasizes several assumptions that are also relevant for the design and interpretation of outcome studies. **First**, the drug abusers can be classified according to differences actually observed in relation to their treatment involvement. This suggests that the universe of drug abusers can be quadrasected, by definition; those who come to treatment and those who do not, and within each, those who make positive changes and those who do not. The natural history or treatment outcomes for these groups reflects their unique composition. For example, those untreated drug abusers who mature out of their addiction lifestyle are simply different people from those who enter treatment and change. This assumption then, avoids the dead end criticism of the non-treatment control since the four groups do not serve as controls for each other.

Treatment effectiveness should be assessed for those clients who seek or perhaps remain in treatment settings. Comparisons involving the clients in the three other groups, however, could reveal much about individual differences and the many influences that contribute to the change process.

Second, client change reflects an interaction between the individual and treatment. This implies mutual, bi-directional influences between the person and the treatment environment. Thus, treatment influences are unique measurable events, are not readily extractable. Futhermore, the global treatment experience itself is an episode, one of many experiences in the individual's continually changing status. Thus, "proving" a treatment influence is less relevant than identifying its particular contribution to a continuing process of individual change.

Third, the primary source of information about this process is the client's own view of the relevant influences. External corroboration of client change through records or other testimony, validates the fact of change, but does not reveal the reason for change. In the last analysis, it is the client who weights the relevant influences in his or her life.

A Perspective on Retention: Dropout is a persistent but perhaps the least understood problem in substance abuse treatment. For therapeutic communities in particular, the importance of retention is illustrated in the fact that research has established a firm relationship between retention and outcome. However, most admissions to therapeutic community programs leave residency, many before treatment influences are presumed to be effectively rendered.

Within the context of the research reviewed, a perspective on retention can be drawn which guides the interpretations of dropout and hypotheses for further research. The drug users who seek treatment, particularly to one modality, are more similar than different. Thus, it is not surprising that research on their social and psychological characteristics reveals relatively low variability, and hence, little power to predict success or retention.

Nevertheless, those who seek treatment could be diverse in ways that have not yet been fully explored. These presumed differences reflect not **who** clients are, in terms of fixed background characteristics, but **how** they perceive themselves, their circumstances and their life options at the time of treatment contact. Assessment of these differences would focus upon at least four domains of client variables which alone or in combination affect dropout. (1) **Circumstances** (extrinsic pressures): These refer to external influences to seek and remain in treatment exerted by family, personal relationships, health and legal conditions, employment, educational and fiscal matters; (2) **Motivation** (intrinsic pressures): This refers to the severity of the problem (felt dissatisfaction, fear, pain) and the expressed need for personal change: (3) **Readiness**: This refers to the perceived need among motivated individuals to elect treatment to assist in personal change compared with non-treatment options, e.g., self-change or religious offerings; (4) **Suitability**: This refers to the client's appropriateness, for, understanding and acceptance of a particular treatment approach.

Treatment Process: The TC cannot improve what it does without clarification of its process. Studies must render explicit the correlation between actual events in treatment and change in client status. It is this interplay between treatment elements and client change which defines process.

The first step in illuminating treatment process is a codification of the TCs perspective, basic elements, assumptions and practices. Several workers have undertaken efforts in this area (see De Leon, 1981; Kerr, Sugarman, Holland & De Leon in this volume).

A next step involves development of program based research capability. Since treatment process research imposes heavy strains on program activities, it is understandably resisted by staff and administration. Thus, acceptance of process studies is facilitated by research teams who know the TC, can integrate with its staff, and can serve in educative roles (De Leon, 1980a).

Alternatives to Long-Term Treatment: Traditional TCs are highly effective for a certain segment of the drug abuse population. However, those who seek assistance in TC settings represent a broad spectrum of clients, most of whom may not be suitable for long-term residential stay, as is evident in the high early dropout rates.

The issue of client diversity underscores the necessity for TCs to develop alternatives to long-term residence and skilled diagnostic-assessment capability. These, however, appear to counter the traditional

TC's open door policy for admissions. Nevertheless, wise assessment of individual differences can only enhance the therapeutic community's capability for retaining those suitable for residential treatment and for offering appropriate options to others who do not enter or stay in long-term treatment. Some TCs have acquired a diagnostic capability, although explicit clinical criteria and appropriate instruments for assessment of client differences remain to be developed.

TCs can offer service alternatives other than long-term residence or referral to other modalities. For example, its method can be modified for both outpatient and short-term residential models. There is an underlying concern that modification could dilute the unique strength of the TC approach itself. Can the traditional TC engineer its social and psychological effects without the 24-hour influence of the residential setting; or, can it maintain the integrity of its community dynamic under a short-term residential regime? These questions remain to be empirically answered. However, the issue of individual differences for the TC need not be one of changing itself, but adapting what it knows and does for the changing client. It is not whether long-term residential treatment is appropriate for all clients; it is clearly not. The task, then is to develop new ways of delivering the basic TC message, and new tactics to produce its unique therapeutic impact.

CHAPTER 8

OUTCOME OF DRUG ABUSE TREATMENT IN TWO MODALITIES

HARRIET BARR

IT IS A generally accepted truism that valid comparisons of the effectiveness of different types of treatment for drug abuse are impossible because the naturally occurring phenomena available for observation do not satisfy criteria for controlled clinical trials. It is not possible to assign drug addicts to treatments randomly, for both practical and ethical reasons. The personal, social and situational conditions that lead a given person to enter one or another form of treatment program have, in fact, the result that clients in different types of programs do differ in many important ways. A strategy such as selecting cases from each of two treatment modalities that are matched on a number of identifiable characteristics does not solve the problem, because the most relevant characteristics — those related to treatment success or failure — are probably not known and not measured.

In spite of these difficulties, this report takes the position that it would be foolish not to examine good treatment outcome data when it is available, that we should find out what can be learned from it, and that caution is necessary in interpreting whatever differences are found. The study on which this report is based has thorough intake data and one year follow-up data on a large sample of drug addicts admitted to two types of treatment, therapeutic community (TC) and methadone maintenance (MM). Only one TC was sampled, as against ten MM programs; if any interpretation is to be made based on program differences, it must therefore be limited to differences between the particular TC studied and the common characteristics of a number of MM programs.

The strategy of analysis has three features. The first is to examine a number of aspects of treatment outcome, on the assumption that each method of treatment is likely to be effective in at least some areas, but that these areas may differ. This approach may identify the relative strengths of each type of treatment. The second is to classify subjects not only by the type of treatment received, but also by the amount of that treatment. The assumption is that better outcome among those receiving more treatment is a necessary (though not sufficient) condition for the demonstration of a treatment effect. The third is to find out whether any of the observed effects can be explained by the pretreatment characteristics of our subjects, rather than by type or amount of treatment.

METHOD

The subjects, instruments and procedures are described in detail elsewhere (Barr & Cohen, 1979) and so will be more briefly summarized here.

Subjects and Follow-Up Rate

The study sample consisted of 866 drug addicts from the greater Philadelphia area first interviewed shortly after admission to treatment and sought for a follow-up interview one year later. The intake interview covered a wide range of aspects of history and status, and revealed them to be a multi-problem treatment population, with adverse family backgrounds and early histories, widespread psychopathology, much criminal justice involvement, and an average of 13 years of drug use. Their average age was 27 years and 27 percent were women; 63 percent were Black, 2 percent Hispanic and the remainder Whites of diverse ethnic origins. Comparison with data from the Central Medical Intake of Philadelphia show this sample to be representative of all drug addicts referred for treatment in the area with regard to demographic characteristics, social background and substance abuse histories.

At the time of follow-up, one year later, 2 percent had died. Follow-up interviews were completed with 90 percent of those living (764 subjects), with no difference in follow-up rate between the TC and MM samples.

Description of Modalities and Definition of Treatment Retention

Since the two types of treatment sampled differ in many important features, including the intended length of treatment, the criteria for treatment retention differ as well.

Methadone Programs (MM). There were 522 subjects followed for the full year, drawn from ten cooperating MM programs in the greater Philadelphia area. All were outpatient programs, with the methadone itself as the major form of therapy, usually combined with an individual counseling session once a week. A minority of clients received other services, such as group therapy (13%), family therapy (7%), or vocational counseling (10%). Some of the programs also offered medical treatment and drop-in recreational facilities.

At the time of follow-up, 31 percent ofthe MM clients had remained in their original programs for the full year, 26 percent had been discharged but on follow-up had been readmitted to the same or a different MM program, 6 percent were in other forms of treatment, and 37 percent were not in treatment. Treatment retention was defined as continuous treatment for the full year. Accordingly, 164 MM subjects were classified as "stayers" and the remaining 358 as "leavers." At the time of follow-up, the "stayers" had therefore received 365 days of MM treatment, and the "leavers" averaged 194 days of treatment in the original programs.

Eagleville (TC). Eagleville Hospital and Rehabilitation Center differ in significant ways from many other TCs. It is a fully accredited hospital, located in a rural setting 28 miles from Philadelphia but serving the entire region, with a staff that includes both professionals with traditional academic training and recovered drug and alcohol addicts (and others) whose training has been less traditional. It treats both drug and alcohol abusers together in a combined program which places strong emphasis on abstinence from all psychoactive substances. The Inpatient Program is an intensive, multimodality two-month residential program. All residents attend at least four group sessions per week and individual sessions as needed, usually one to three times per week. There are regular community and unit meetings, activities, occupational therapy, educational and work therapy programs.

Of those who successfully complete the Inpatient Program, 40-45 percent remain on the hospital grounds for a transitional work and therapy program known as the Candidate Program, lasting up to six months.

Of the TC subjects followed, 22 percent had completed the inpatient phase and participated in the Candidate Program, with an average of 172 days of residential treatment, and 31 percent had left residential treatment after completing the inpatient phase, with an average of 54 days stay. These two groups, consisting of 129 subjects, were classified as "stayers," and they averaged 102 days of residential treatment. The remaining 113 residents left against medical advice, eloped or were discharged for violations of rules after an average of 32 days, and were classified as "leavers."

Outcome Measures

Ten outcome measures were examined, covering five areas of functioning: alcohol use and abuse, drug use and abuse, dysphoria, criminal justice involvement, and employment. Each was measured both prior to entering treatment and at the time of follow-up, with different time frames for different measures. Follow-up status on each of the outcome measures was, to some degree, correlated with pre-treatment status on the corresponding measure or measures; the pre-post r's (or R's) ranged from .208 to .451. In order to obtain a purer measure of treatment effect, the influence of each subject's status on the appropriate pre-treatment covariate or covariates was partialled out of each outcome measure. The resulting residual scores, which were used in all analyses, were than standardized for each of comparison.

Analyses of the outcome measures of alcohol and drug use and abuse are based on a reduced sample of 658 subjects who were at risk for substance use, omitting 106 subjects who were in prison when interviewed at one year. Analyses of nonsubstance use measures are based on the full sample of 764 cases.

The outcome measures and their pre-treatment covariances are:

1. **Alcohol consumption** for the two months preceding follow-up is based on a quantity-frequency measure of the average amount of absolute alcohol consumed daily, summed for liquor, beer and wine, and submitted to a logarithmic transformation (covariates: alcohol consumption in the two months prior to intake; alcohol consumption during the period when the subject's drinking was greatest).

2. **Alcohol-related problems** during the two months preceding follow-up is a weighted sum of reported loss of control over drinking, bad reactions to alcohol, negative life consequences from drinking, and drunkeness (covariates: alcohol-related problems in the two months prior to intake; lifetime history of alcohol-related problems).

3. **Motivation for drinking** is a scale of items reporting positive benefits given either as reasons for drinking or gains experienced by the respondent. Examples are: to forget your worries; feel happy, relaxed; have fun; relief from anxiety, pain, tension; relate better to people (covariate; pre-treatment motivation for drinking).

4. The **drug use index** is a scale that takes into account all classes of drugs used. It gives greater weight to regular use than to irregular use, and less weight to marijuana than to other drugs. Drugs used only as prescribed are not counted (covariates: number of drug categories used at all and number of drug categories used regularly in the two months before intake).

5. **Drug-related problems** is a weighted score based on loss of control over drug use, bad reactions to drugs and negative life consequences from drug use (covariate: the intake measure is based on the lifetime history of drug problems).

6. **Motivation for drug use** is directly parallel to the analogous alcohol measure (covariate: pre-treatment motivation for gains from drug use).

7. **Dysphoria** is an 18-item scale of feelings and symptoms during the past two months; it is the sum of three highly intercorrelated self-report scales: depression, phobic anxiety, and happiness (sign reversed) (covariate: dysphoria in the two months before intake).

8. **Criminal justice involvement** is an index based on number of arrests, number of convictions and time spent in prison during the year of follow-up (covariates: lifetime number of arrests, number of convictions and time spent in prison).

9. **Months (un)employed** during the year of follow-up is based on all paid employment, including that of TC subjects while in the candidate program and MM subjects in work training programs. It does not compensate for the fact that TC subjects were unavailable for employment during their stay as inpatients (covariates: months worked in the two years prior to intake; employment status on intake as defined below).

10. **Employment status** at the time of follow-up gives full weight to full-time employment, and partial weight to part-time employment, school and homemaking (covariates: months worked in the two months prior to intake; employment status on intake).

Method of Analysis

Two-way analyses of variance (ANOVA) were performed for each outcome measure, with treatment retention (stay vs. leaving) and modality (TC vs. MM) as the independent variables, making it possible to assess each main effect independently as well as their interaction.

Following this, each outcome measure was further controlled by partialling out the influence of those aspects of the intake history most strongly correlated with it. This precedure tests whether the significant findings of the ANOVAs can be readily explained by pre-treatment differences among subjects.

Analysis of Variance: Effects of Retention and Modality

Significant effects occurred by modality and treatment retention. The strongest determinant of outcome, overall, is staying in treatment, which has a significant (.01 or .001 level) main effect on all seven non-alcohol outcome measures. For each of these outcome measures the difference between "stayers" and "leavers" is in the same direction for both the Eagleville and methadone samples and there is no interaction effect.

For four of these outcome measures there is also a significant main effect for treatment modality, although in each case it is smaller than that for retention. Eagleville subjects had better outcomes in regard to drug use, motivation for drug use and months worked, and they had much worse outcomes in the criminal justice area. These differences will be examined further below.

The three measures of involvement with alcohol show a different pattern. The significant effect in this area is the interaction of modality and retention; those who completed the Eagleville inpatient program have the best outcomes, while the other three groups do not differ significantly. There are no significant main effects for modality, and the one significant main effect for retention, that for motivation for drinking, is entirely due to the strong effect among the Eagleville subjects, since methadone subjects show a negligible difference in the opposite direction.

We may therefore conclude that a longer stay in methadone maintenance programs does not reduce drug addicts' involvement with alcohol, while completion of inpatient treatment at Eagleville is associated with a significant reduction in drinking and related problems, as well as in motivation for drinking.

Can Pre-Treatment Differences Explain The Findings?

The significant main effects for treatment modality on four of the outcome measures must be viewed with great suspicion, since we have violated the classical experimental rule of random assignment of subjects to treatments. To be sure, each outcome measure was controlled for each subject's status on the corresponding measure or measures obtained at the time of intake. The pre-treatment convariates, however, account for only between 4 percent and 20 percent of the variance in the different aspects of outcome.

Do client differences account for treatment retention as well? Although evidence of better outcomes among those who stay in treatment has a more obvious face validity than evidence of modality differences in outcome, the findings do not prove such effects in any scientific sense, since experimental control over treatment retention is also lacking. Whether a client stays in treatment or leaves prematurely is surely determined to a substantial extent by the person's past history and present condition on admission to treatment, as well as by what happens during treatment and the interaction between person and treatment.

An attempt was made to control for pre-treatment differences among subjects statistically. The control variables were derived from the extensive intake interview held with each subject shortly after admission to treatment. A set of 54 variables was available, covering demographic data, family background, childhood and school history, work history, criminal justice history, a thorough lifetime and current drug and alcohol history, and psychological self-report scales. From one to three of these measures served as the pre-test covariate or covariates for each outcome measure. Of the remaining 51 to 53 intake measures, the four with the highest r's with each outcome measure were used as control for that measure.

The first step in the procedure was to use multiple regression analysis to compute the mean outcome score that would be predicted for each subgroup of subjects on the basis of its scores for the four control variables. For example, the four best intake predictors of motivation for drug use on follow-up, after pretreatment motivation for drug use is partialled out, are dysphoria, having few close friends, disciplinary problems in school, and alienation. The outcome status predicted by these variables was subtracted from the actual outcome score, providing a measure of the residual unexplained variance in the outcome measure. The modality/retention subgroups were then compared with regard to that residual score.

Retention. The controls had no effect on the relationships with treatment retention. For none of the outcome measures did they account for an appreciable portion of the difference between stayers and leavers, all p-values for retention were unchanged.

Modality. Of the four outcome measures for which there was a significant main effect of treatment modality, two were substantially explained by the intake control measures and two were not. Controlling for intake characteristics did not affect the six outcome measures that did not have a significant modality effect originally.

The two aspects of outcome that were explained to a substantial degree were criminal justice involvement and months not working. Of the eleven intake variables that were significantly related ($p < .01$ or $.001$) to criminal justice involvement on follow-up, nine also differentiated at the $.001$ level between the Eagleville and methadone samples. In all nine, the direction associated with greater criminal justice involvement characterized the Eagleville sample. Seven intake measures were related to unemployment at the $.05$ level or less; for all seven, the direction associated with less employment was more typical of methadone subjects, significantly so for four of them.

Thus, the greater criminal involvement on follow-up of Eagleville subjects and the greater unemployment of methadone subjects cannot be interpreted as evidence of differences in effectiveness between the two types of treatment programs, but rather as a reflection of differences in the types of clients each admits. In contrast, controlling for pretreatment characteristics did not reduce the relationships between modality and either drug use or motivation for drug use. The biserial r for modality with drug use rose from $.103$ to $.124$, and that with motivation for drug use rose from $.107$ to $.119$ ($516.$ at the $.01$ level). This reflects the fact that the intake correlates of these two outcome measures were not found to characterize the clients of either modality consistently.

Finally, the significant interaction effects of retention and modality on the three alcohol outcome measures were unchanged when additional intake variables were controlled for.

Summary of Findings

Analysis of the effects of treatment retention and modality on ten aspects of drug abuse treatment outcome at one year, controlling for intake characteristics, showed that:

1. For three measure of alcohol use and abuse there was a significant interaction effect, i.e., staying in treatment was associated with better outcomes for Eagleville residents, but not for methadone maintenance clients.

2. For three measures of drug use and abuse there was a highly significant association between treatment retention and better outcome, regardless of modality. There was a smaller but significant finding that Eagleville subjects had better outcomes with regard to drug use and motivation for drug use; there was no modality difference in drug related problems. Controlling for certain intake variables did not alter these findings.

3. Four measures of non-substance use aspects of outcome — dysphoria, criminal justice involvement, and two measures of employment — were all significantly related in the expected direction to treatment retention, regardless of modality. Two of these measures also showed significant modality differences. Outcomes were better among methadone clients in the criminal justice area, and they were better among Eagleville subjects with regard to the number of months of employment. However, controlling for relevant intake characteristics of subjects eliminated the significant modality effects, but did not change the associations between staying in treatment and better outcomes.

DISCUSSION

The findings confirm the effectiveness of two types of treatment for drug abuse by demonstrating that, for both modalities, drug addicts who have received more treatment have significantly better outcomes than those who have left treatment prematurely. The superior outcomes of those who have had more treatment can be observed in their substance abuse and in other aspects of functioning as well. Unanswered is the philosophical question of the extent to which this is "caused by" the treatment or is the result of the individual's readiness of change — possibly in some cases a readiness to change that would have been effective without treatment. In that sense, the effectiveness of treatment, per se, can probably never be demonstrated. Nevertheless, the evidence is clear that those drug addicts who can and do avail themselves of treatment, for whatever reasons, are much more successfully rehabilitated than those who do not.

Although the magnitude of the treatment effect (i.e., the mean difference between "stayers" and "leavers") varies across the outcome measures for each modality, the average treatment effect for the seven drug and nonsubstance abuse aspects of outcome (temporarily ignoring the alcohol measures) is remarkably similar for the TC and MM samples, amounting to .4. This is perhaps surprising in view of the many differences between the two modalities. Treatment retention in the MM programs represents a much longer course of treatment; TC treatment is, however, much more intensive and comprehensive. Furthermore, a larger proportion of TC subjects than MM subjects satisfied program requirements for treatment stay (53 vs. 31). There is some evidence in the present sample that matching of client to type of treatment is significantly better than chance, although admittedly very far from perfect. We may venture the hypothesis that, if a drug addict enters a type of treatment that meets his or her needs and is able to stick with that treatment, the average level of treatment gain will be similar in spite of differences among different types of drug addicts and the particular forms of treatment best suited to each.

The differences that were found between methadone clients and ex-residents of the one TC that was sampled must be examined in the light of the nature of each type of program. These differences are entirely in the measures of substance use and involvement, since the modality effects observed in other areas were readily explained by the types of patients each treats.

The clearest difference was that completion of treatment at Eagleville produced significant reduction in motivation for drinking, actual alcohol consumption and alcohol-related problems, while methadone treatment did not. The interaction effects between modality and retention found for the drinking measures are probably the most robust evidence possible of a modality difference in effectiveness.

The explanation probably lies in the generic nature of the Eagleville program. Abusers of drugs and of alcohol are treated together in a completely integrated combined treatment program; at any one time, 50 percent to 60 percent of the residents have a primary diagnosis of alcoholism. There is a strong emphasis on the goal of abstinence from all psychoactive substances for all residents, regardless of the particular substance or substances they may have abused before entering treatment. Both drug addicts and alcoholics attend meetings of Alcoholics Anonymous and Narcotics Anonymous during their stay at Eagleville, and drug addicts as well as alcoholics often choose to take antabuse to help maintain their sobriety.

In contrast, methadone programs are explicitly aimed at the reduction of narcotic use. While alcohol abuse is likely to be recognized as a problem when it becomes very obvious, MM programs vary greatly in their sensitivity to alcohol problems and their ability to deal with them.

All too often, treatment staff are ill-equipped to recognize the early stages of alcoholism in their clients and they are likely to lack training in dealing with it. Furthermore, the message conveyed by a methadone program is not one of abstinence. In regard to drug use, the message is rather that "you should take the narcotic we prescribe and give you daily, and you should stop using illicit drugs." Such a message does not, in itself, discourage the use of the legal drug alcohol.

Thus, abstinence from alcohol is a major treatment goal for drug addicts at Eagleville, but not in the typical methadone maintenance program, and our findings demonstrate that the differences in goals is reflected in a difference in outcomes. Evidence that this is an important goal in the rehabilitation of drug addicts is found not only in our own work (Barr & Cohen, 1979), but in the work of other investigators as well (e.g., De Leon, 1984; Simpson & Sells, 1982; Des Jarlais, Joseph & Dole, 1981). It has been well established that alcohol abuse is a complicating problem in a substantial minority of drug addicts, and that its presence creates a significant interference with both treatment and the prospects for successful rehabilitation. Alcoholism has been reported as a major problem in methadone treatment programs. The findings of this study suggest that it is essential to obtain thorough alcohol histories from drug addicts being referred for treatment, so that those for whom drinking is a past, present or potential problem can be placed in a treatment program that is designed to deal with the abuse of alcohol as well as abuse of other drugs. Methadone maintenance is not the treatment of choice for the drug addict who is also a problem drinker.

Two of the drug abuse variables — drug use and motivation for drug use — showed a significant main effect, with better outcomes among Eagleville subjects; no such effect was found with regard to drug-related problems. The three measures may be viewed (with great oversimplification) as representing three phases in the development of drug abuse, with corresponding stages that must be gone through in recovery from drug abuse. First drugs are tried, then positive effects are experienced leading to increased use of drugs; then the problems and negative effects develop, often leading to continued or increased use of drugs in an attempt to overcome them and to recapture the previously experienced benefits. If there is a difference in the effectiveness of the TC and MM programs in the drug area, it appears reasonable that such an effect would be seen in regard to drug motivation and use before it would affect drug problems.

This line of reasoning is admittedly speculative, and the evidence for a modality difference in treating the drug abuse of our subjects must be considered tentative at best. In the intake interview, Eagleville residents reported significantly higher levels of drug motivation than did MM clients. Their actual levels of drug motivation on follow-up were not significantly different; rather, their motivation for drug use on follow-up represented a greater decrease from pre-treatment levels.

This does not apply to the difference in drug use on follow-up, which was significantly less among Eagleville subjects regardless of whether pre-treatment levels are taken into account, a finding not related to treatment retention. TC leavers reported significantly ($p <$ .05) less drug use on follow-up than did MM leavers.

The finding that requires explanation is, then, the relatively low level of drug use among those who did not complete treatment at Eagleville. On follow-up, this group reported continuing high levels of motivation for drug use and drug-related problems, in a setting of reduced drug use. Any interpretation of this phenomenon must be offered most tentatively. It is possible that the strong abstinence ethic promoted by the Eagleville program reaches at least some of those who remain in treatment for only a short time. Without the benefit of the full program, however, there is little impact on the addict's psychological investment in drug use or the problems created by it. One might speculate that, therefore, for this group, reduction in drug use will be short-lived unless there is a return to some form of treatment. (The importance of psychological changes during treatment and the stability of outcome in TC's has been reported in other studies, e.g., De Leon, 1984; Biase, 1982.)

In conclusion, the data reported here show that drug addicts who fulfill the program's goal for treatment retention in either methadone maintenance or the one TC that was studied have better outcomes than other addicts in regard to drug abuse, dysphoria, criminal justice involvement and employment. Involvement with alcohol and alcohol-related problems among these drug addicts were not reduced by methadone treatment, but were significantly reduced by treatment in an abstinence-oriented TC that treats alcohol and drug abusers in a combined treatment program.

CHAPTER 9

12-YEAR FOLLOW-UP OUTCOMES OF OPIOID ADDICTS TREATED IN THERAPEUTIC COMMUNITIES

D. DWAYNE SIMPSON

A S THE ACCOMPANYING papers in this book demonstrate, the TC treatment research literature has grown in size and sophistication over the past 15 years. The general effectiveness of this treatment has been documented (De Leon, 1984; Simpson & Sells, 1982; Tims & Ludford, 1984), but more research is needed which focuses on details of the therapeutic process. In addition, relatively little is known about the long-term outcomes of clients admitted to TC programs because of the short history of community-based drug abuse treatments.

In 1969, the Drug Abuse Reporting Program (DARP) began collecting admission and during-treatment records on clients entering therapeutic communities (TCs) and other major treatment modalities provided by community-based agencies located across the United States. The DARP served as a basis for extensive research on client characteristics, treatment classifications, and during-treatment performance (Sells, 1974; Sells & Simpson, 1976), and this data base has been used for 6-year post-DARP follow-up research on treatment effectiveness (Simpson & Sells, 1982; Simpson, in press) and most

This work was supported by the National Institute on Drug Abuse grant DA03419 as part of the longitudinal research project which began in 1968. The interpretations and conclusions, however, do not necessarily represent the position of NIDA or the Department of Health and Human Services.

Appreciation is expressed to Wayne Lehman, and Kerry Marsh for assisting with data analysis, and to George Joe for editorial comments.

109

effectiveness (Simpson & Sells, 1982; Simpson, in press) and most recently for 12-year follow-up research on addiction careers. This paper summarizes some early results from the 12-year follow-up of opioid addicts admitted to DARP treatments, giving particular attention to clients of TC programs.

METHOD

Sample

Admissions to DARP drug abuse treatment programs totaled 27,214 during the period of June 1969 through May 1972. From this population base, a stratified random sample of 4,107 clients from 25 different DARP agencies located across the United States was selected for the 6-year follow-up study (Simpson & Joe, 1977); 87 percent of the cases were located, and successful interviews were completed with 3,131 respondents. The stratification factors included DARP treatment classification, time in treatment, race-ethnic group, sex, age, and treatment agency or clinic. The follow-up sample included clients from methadone maintenance (MM) programs, therapeutic communities (TC), outpatient drug-free treatments (DF), outpatient detoxification (DT), and an intake only (IO) group whose members completed intake and admission procedures but did not return for treatment in DARP.

From the completed 6-year interviews, a total of 697 persons were selected for a 12-year follow-up study of opioid addiction careers. All were daily opioid users at the time of DARP admission. They were drawn from 18 different DARP treatment agencies, as explained in more detail by Simpson (1984a). The fieldwork, including locating and interviewing the sample, was carried out during 1982 and 1983 by the National Opinion Research Center (NORC) under a subcontract. In summary, 80 percent of the target sample were located; 490 (70%) were interviewed after granting informed consent, 52 (8%) were deceased, and 13 (2%) refused to be interviewed. The remaining 142 (20%) were not located before time and resources for the fieldwork ran out. Analysis of DARP admissions and 6-year follow-up data, however, revealed no evidence of sampling bias associated with the nonlocated cases (Simpson, 1984a).

Follow-up interviews were conducted face-to-face by trained interviewers following strict procedures to protect the confidentiality of data. The average duration of each interview was approximately 2 hours, for which the respondent was paid $15. The interview focused on behavioral changes and outcomes over time, as well as historical assessments of psychological and social factors involved throughout the addiction career. Major criterion behaviors included illicit drug use, drug abuse treatment, alcohol use, employment, and criminality. Checks for internal consistency, as well as comparisons of self-reported information with results of urinanalyses and with criminal justice records of post-DARP incarcerations, indicated a high level of reliability and validity of the data (Simpson, 1984b).

Therapeutic Community Sample. The present study focuses on outcomes for the subsample of addicts who were admitted to TCs in the DARP. Out of 135 black and white males selected from TC programs for the 12-year follow-up study, 99 (73%) were interviewed, 10 (8%) were deceased, and 26 (19%) were not located. The interviewed sample represented 12 different treatment agencies, ranging from 3 to 12 per agency, and were evenly represented by Blacks (n = 52) and Whites (n = 47). With regard to age, 14 percent were 26 to 30 years old, 52 percent were 31 to 35, 23 percent were 36 to 40, and 11 percent were over 40 at the time of the follow-up interview. Forty-three percent were currently married (or living as married), 36 percent were divorced or separated, 1 percent were widowed, and 20 percent had never been married; 35 percent had been married two or more times, and 70 percent had children.

RESULTS

Tabulations were made of behavioral criteria for time periods representing the pre-DARP baseline through the 12-year DARP follow-up interview. The 6-year follow-up study gathered information on a retrospective basis from termination of DARP treatment until the year 6 follow-up interviews. Thus, it served as the basis for outcome tabulations in years 1 to 3 immediately after termination of DARP treatment and year 6 following admission to DARP. The 12-year follow-up study served as the basis for outcome tabulations in year 12 following admission to DARP. (It should be pointed out that the calendar dates for years 1, 2, and 3 post-DARP data were differentially determined by the length of time each particular respondent spent in DARP treatment. Therefore, the amount of time between the year 3 and year 6 data was actually less than 3 years for persons who remained in DARP treatment for a year or longer.) Except for incarceration in jail or prison, tabulations in each time period were based only on persons who spent time "at risk" (i.e., those not confined in jail or other residential treatment facilities for entire time).

Stability of Outcomes Over Time

Drug use was grouped into three categories: opioids (heroin, illegal methadone, and other opiates), marijuana, and other nonopioids (cocaine, amphetamines/stimulants, barbiturates/sedatives, and hallucinogens). Table 1 shows that opioid use by this sample of former TC addicts dropped to 52 percent in year 1 after DARP treatment (including 38% who used daily during 1 or more months that year) and to 34 percent in year 12 following DARP admission (including 23% who used daily during 1 or more months that year). This opioid use primarily involved heroin, and in some cases more than one opioid drug was used. Marijuana use remained relatively stable over the 12-year period, but with a high of 62 percent who used in year 12. Other nonopioid drugs were used by 62 percent before DARP admission, followed by a low of 31 percent in year 1 and back up to 43 percent in year 12. (Further inspection of these data revealed that the increase in nonopioid use during the post-DARP follow-up period was explained by an apparent upsurge in cocaine use.)

Treatment for drug use dropped to a low of 29 percent in year 12, which was consistent with the drop in opioid use throughout the follow-up period. The alcohol consumption data show there was an increase in alcohol use (measured in 80-proof liquor equivalent) after DARP, followed by a steady decline in use over the follow-up period back to a level near or just below pre-DARP levels. Among those who had quit daily opioid use, 25 percent said they had previously used alcohol as a substitute in place of opioid drugs while quitting. In year 12, 20 percent of the sample drank an average of over 4 ounces per day (including 10% who drank over 8 ounces per day), and other data revealed that 13 percent reported they received treatment for alcohol use that year. Together, these data indicate that while average alcohol consumption increased and opioid use dropped from immediately before to after DARP treatment, this trend of apparent alcohol substitution did not continue throughout the follow-up periods when opioid and alcohol use both continued to decrease.

For criminal involvement, pre-DARP baseline data were available only for lifetime arrest and incarceration rates. While limiting compari-

Table 1

SUMMARY OF BEHAVIORAL OUTCOME
MEASURES OVER TIME (N=99)

Outcome Measures	Pre-DARP	Post-DARP Follow-up				
		Year 1	Year 2	Year 3	6th Year	12th Year
DRUG USE:						
% Daily opioids	100	38	28	26	21	23
% Any opioids	100	52	41	36	33	34
% Any marijuana	54	55	57	53	60	62
% Any other non-opioids	62	31	32	38	39	43
DRUG TREATMENT:						
% 1 or more times	62	30	32	32	33	29
ALCOHOL USE (in 80-proof):						
% Over 4 oz/day	22	33	26	24	24	20
% Over 8 oz/day	14	16	12	13	12	10
CRIMINAL INVOLVEMENT:						
% Any arrests	99	27	24	17	19	11
% Any jail or prison	66	29	33	30	27	30
EMPLOYMENT:						
% 1 or more months	66	77	77	82	84	78
% 6 or more months	32	61	69	71	72	60

Note. For pre-DARP measures, drug and alcohol use was based on the last 2 months before admission to DARP, employment was based on the last 12 months, and drug treatment and criminality were lifetime measures. Sample sizes were adjusted in each time period so that tabulations were based only on persons who were "at risk" (e.g., persons in jail during an entire year were omitted from drug use and employment tabulations for that period).

sons with post-DARP follow-up periods, these data show that almost the entire sample had criminal histories — 99 percent had been arrested and 88 percent jailed. After DARP, arrest rates (based each year on persons with 1 or more months at risk) declined from 27 percent in year 1 to 11 percent in year 12, while incarceration rates (based on the total sample) remained stable at about 30 percent from years 1 to 12.

The percentage of the sample employed in 1 or more months each year from pre-DARP baseline to the 12-year follow-up ranged from 66 percent to 84 percent, and persons who worked in 6 or more months (or 50% or more of the months at risk) during each of these years ranged from 32 percent to 72 percent of the sample. Employment rates were highest in year 6; they declined in year 12, when 78 percent reported any employment and 60 percent worked in 6 or more months.

Composite Outcomes in Year 12

Since several different behavioral criteria are important to consider in assessing follow-up outcomes of former addicts, individual measures have been combined in various ways in the DARP research to form composites. Outcomes on six major behavioral measures were also categorized using two separate criterion definitions. These measures included opioid drug use, nonopioid drug use, criminality, reentry to drug treatment, alcohol use, and employment. Each of these six criteria was examined both individually and as part of a composite profile that represents a more comprehensive view of behavioral performance by using a sequential approach to the classification of individual status as developed in previous work by Bracy and Simpson (1982-83). Two separate criterion standards were used — Highly Favorable Standards and Moderately Favorable Standards.

For the **highly favorable** standard, the individual outcome criteria specified (1) no opioid use, (2) no nonopioid use (except for less-than daily marijuana use), (3) no criminality, (4) no drug treatment, (5) low alcohol use, and (6) high employment during the last year before the follow-up interview. "No criminality" was defined as no arrests and no incarcerations in the last year before the follow-up interview. "Low alcohol use" referred to average daily use of less than 4 oz. of 80-proof liquor equivalent, and "high employment" referred to working in 6 or more months (or 50% or more of the months while at risk) during the last year.

Criterion specifications for the **moderately favorable** standard included (1) no daily opioid use, (2) no daily nonopioid use, (3) no major criminality, (4) no drug treatment, (5) no heavy alcohol use, and (6) some employment during the last year. "Major criminality" was defined as 30 days or more in jail or prison during the last year, or any arrests for crimes against persons (e.g., murder, assault) or crimes of profit (e.g., robbery, burglary). Thus, short periods of incarceration or arrests for "victimless" crimes (such as prostitution and gambling) were not considered to reflect major criminal involvement. "No heavy alcohol use" meant less than 8 oz. of 80-proof alcohol per day, and "some employment" meant working in any 1 or more months during the last year.

A third of the sample (32%) reported no drug use as well as no arrests or jail. And finally, 21 percent met all six criteria, indicating no drug use, no criminality, no treatment, low alcohol use, and 6 months or more of employment. For the moderately favorable outcome conditions, almost one-half of the sample (46%) met the major criteria of no daily drug use and no major criminality, while 32 percent met all six criterion.

Reasons for Starting Addiction

When asked, "In your own words, what do you think was the main reason you ever got started using opiate drugs daily?" 61 percent of the follow-up sample mentioned the influence of peers, 32 percent referred to escape from boredom or problems, 20 percent noted their curiosity, 15 percent said they liked the good feelings from opioids, and smaller percentages reported a variety of other reasons. This question was then followed by a list of specific reasons developed from the research literature on addiction, and respondents were asked to rate the importance of each one as a reason for why they first began daily opioid use. This rating involved a 4-point scale — very important, somewhat important, not too important, and not important at all.

The major reasons given in response to the open-ended question about starting addiction were generally represented in the prepared list of specific reasons. The items receiving the highest percentage of "very important" ratings involved the immediate physiological and psychological effects of the drug — relaxation (70%), euphoric rush (69%), and escape by forgetting troubles (61%). These reasons were almost universally endorsed as being important. Next was the excitement of drug use (42%), followed by its easy availability (32%).

It is interesting to note that the relative importance attached to these reasons appeared to have differed between the two response formats. For instance, the influence of peers was reflected in the cluster of **interpersonal** reasons including pressure from close friends, showing defiance, emulation of (or trying to be like) persons who used drugs, and using drugs to impress others (or showing toughness "on the street"). However, these items received lower overall ratings than did **environmental** and **intraindividual** reasons. About half of the sample considered pressure from close friends, emulation of other users, and efforts to impress others to be "very" or "somewhat" important reasons for starting addiction, but 67 percent to 98 percent gave similar ratings to availability, sensation-seeking, euphoria, and anxiety reduction. Medical use and showing independence from family were given the lowest ratings.

Length of Addiction

The age at last daily opioid use was under 20 years for 6 percent of the sample, 20 to 24 years for 25 percent, 25 to 29 years for 32 percent, 30 to 34 years for 26 percent, and 35 years or older for 11 percent. As already noted, 23 percent used opioid drugs daily during 1 or more months of year 12 after admission to DARP TC treatment. Thus, the overall length of opioid addiction for these particular indviduals was still undefined at the time of the follow-up interview. Calculations of the length of time between the first daily opioid use and last use (or the time of interview if opioids had been used daily in year 12) showed that 27 percent had 1 to 5 years of addiction, 28 percent had 5 to 10 years, 38 percent had 10 to 20 years, and 6 percent had over 20 years. The median was 9.4 years.

Three-fourths of the sample said they had quit daily opioid use at least once and then later relapsed. Although half the sample was addicted 9.4 years or longer, only 34 percent ever had a period of continuous daily use which exceeded 2 years (24 percent reported having continuous addiction periods which lasted more than 3 years).

Reasons for Continued Use and Quitting Addiction

The findings indicate that motivations for opioid use change over the course of addiction careers. Comparisons of reasons for opioid use during the **last addiction period** with those for first starting daily use showed that the majority of addicts continued to consider drug availability as well as the euphoric and anxiety reduction effects of opioid drugs as important motivations for use. However, ratings dropped over this time for sensation-seeking motivations for interpersonal influences; for example, "very important" and "somewhat important" ratings from the first to the last daily use decreased from 90 percent to 10 percent for sensation-seeking, 44 percent to 17 percent for pressure from close friends, 28 percent to 8 percent for showing defiance toward family and others, 53 percent to 10 percent for emulation of other users, and 45 percent to 6 percent for impressing others (see Joe & Chastain, 1984, for detailed analysis of these data).

By year 12, three-fourths of the sample had been abstinent for a year or longer. When asked "In your own words, what were the main reasons why you quit using opiate drugs daily the last time?" 62 percent said they became tired of the life, 39 percent stated a fear of the law (e.g., jail, prison, or parole violation), and 18 percent acknowledged the influence of family or friends. Several other reasons — such as drug cost or financial problems, drug quality or availability, health problems, fear of overdose or death, and accessibility of treatment — were each mentioned by fewer than 10 percent of the sample. In response to a similar question about quitting, 64 percent said it occurred as a result of a deliberate decision to do so, while 28 percent felt that it just seemed to happen as a result of life changes in which drug use became less important.

Responses to a list of specific reasons for quitting addiction were obtained with an open-ended question. The most frequent reasons involved **psychological** and **emotional** problems. These were characterized by being tired of the hustle (rated as "very" or "somewhat" important by 81% of the sample) and needing a change after "hitting bottom" (72%). These reasons were followed in level of importance by fear of being sent to jail (62%), other "personal or special" influential events (59%), and the need to meet family responsibilities (45%).

Drug Abuse Treatments

Ninety-seven percent of the sample reported receiving treatment specifically for their opioid use. Overall, 11 percent had been in a TC program three or more times. The majority had been in methadone maintenance programs (64%, and 18% had been in three or more times) and detoxification-only programs (57%, and 20% had been in three or more times), while 38 percent had been in outpatient drug-free programs (4% for three or more times).

The major reasons rated as important for going into treatment programs included making a personal decision of wanting treatment (85%), the influence of a spouse or other family member (77%), legal referrals (59%), and pressure from a parole or probation officer (45%). Almost three-fourths of the sample (71%) indicated that they had quit opioid drug use "as a result of treatment." The aspects of treatment programs named as "most helpful" were the counseling services (48%) and the opportunities treatment provided for reflection and making personal decisions about drug use (35%). Also, the use of methadone as part of treatment was approved by 57 percent of the sample.

Among persons who had no daily opioid use during the last year or longer before the follow-up interview, 65 percent were in some type of treatment when they quit; of this subsample that was in treatment, 42 percent were in a TC and 36 percent were in methadone maintenance. Almost a third admitted using another drug (usually alcohol) as a substitute when they quit opioid use. Avoidance of old friends, hangouts, and social settings, along with the development of new friendships, work habits, and family ties were considered important in maintaining abstinence.

SUMMARY AND CONCLUSIONS

Drug use, criminality, and employment outcomes improved for opioid addicts from before to after treatment in DARP TC programs, and other studies have shown these improvements had positive relationships with the length of the time spent in treatment (Simpson 1979, 1981) and the occurrence of other treatment episodes after DARP (Simpson & Savage, 1980). Studies of other TC programs have shown similiar results (De Leon, 1984). Post-DARP follow-up data have also demonstrated that MM, TC, and DF programs had more favorable posttreatment outcomes than did comparison groups of detoxification and intake-only clients (Simpson, Savage, & Lloyd, 1979; Simpson & Sells, 1982). It is of importance, therefore, that the 12-year retrospective evaluations of treatments by former clients support these findings on treatment effectiveness; that is, the majority of former addicts in this study (65%) reported being in treatment at the time they quit daily opioid use, and they credited treatment services as being a major factor in helping them to quit.

Comparisons between the 6-year and 12-year follow-up outcomes show that overall behavioral measures remained stable without major improvements over this time period. As reported by Simpson, Joe, Lehman, Sells (in press), client outcomes were generally consistent between years 6 to 12, but most of the standard pre-DARP background and demographic measures proved to be poor predictors of long-term outcomes (Lehman & Caillouet, 1984). Additional DARP research examining addiction careers and follow-up outcomes in relation to childhood relations with family and peers as well as psychological adjustment are being examined, although the behaviorally-oriented DARP data base is limited in the availability of psychological measures which can be examined for this purpose.

The median length of addiction careers in the 12-year follow-up data for former TC clients was 9.4 years, but only one-fourth of the sample reported ever having a continuous "run" of daily opioid use which lasted over 3 years. Three-fourths had quit and then later relapsed to daily use one or more times, usually due to craving the pleasurable physical and psychological effects of opioids. The relapse rate is indicative of the highly cyclical nature of addiction careers and deserves further study. At the time of the 12-year follow-up interview, 23 percent of the sample still used opioid drugs daily, but almost half (46%) had no daily use of any illicit drugs and no major criminal involvement in the previous years.

In addition to the relaxing and anxiety-reducing effects of opioid drugs, social and peer influences were found to be the most important reasons for initially becoming addicted. These social and interpersonal factors lost their significance over time, however, and the psychological properties attributed to opioids (i.e., the euphoria and anxiety-reduction) were the major reasons for sustained use — and for relapses after temporary abstinence. Termination of addiction was most often motivated by psychological and emotional crises in which the addict "hit bottom" and decided to change. A variety of special events appeared to be involved in reaching this decision stage, but it was interesting to find legal influences (particularly the fear of being incarcerated) as one of the major considerations.

The present study focused on a sample of TC clients, but as Simpson et al., (in press) pointed out in a similar study based on the combined DARP treatment samples, long-term follow-up outcomes were not significantly related to the original DARP treatment assignments. Even though a client's treatment history may be associated with some addiction career differences (such as an increased role for legal referrals and influences among TC clients), reasons for starting and quitting addiction involved minimal differences between TC and other DARP treatment groups. It must be recognized, however, that over the course of their addiction careers most individuals in the present follow-up sample were exposed to a variety of treatments. Thus, there are very few "pure" treatment clients who can be identified in most long-term follow-up research.

Based on previous results from the 6-year DARP follow-up studies, a major unexpected finding in the 12-year data was the leveling off of "favorable" outcomes between years 6 and 12. Since daily opioid use dropped by about 75 percent from pre-DARP to the 6-year follow-up, of course, the range allowed for further improvements became more restricted after year 6. Indeed, there probably are additional limitations which should be imposed on expected improvements because of the socioeconomic level and environmental settings which are characteristic of most of these former DARP treatment clients. Since almost half of the sample maintained opioid abstinence in both years 6 and 12, while the other half was evenly split between those who increased and those who decreased their use over time, these different outcome groups need to be explored in more detail.

CHAPTER 10

DAYTOP MINIVERSITY — PHASE 2 COLLEGE TRAINING IN A THERAPEUTIC COMMUNITY — DEVELOPMENT OF SELF CONCEPT AMONG DRUG FREE ADDICT/ABUSERS

D. VINCENT BIASE

ARTHUR P. SULLIVAN

BARBARA WHEELER

DAYTOP MINIVERSITY, funded in part by the National Institute on Drug Abuse is a research demonstration project applicable to the advancement of drug rehabilitation and college level education. The Project begun in February 1979 has successfully demonstrated and empirically evaluated the deployment of a three semester matriculated college program within a major drug-free therapeutic community. The subjects are identified addicts or poly drug abusers undergoing drug-free residential treatment and rehabilitation within Daytop Village, New York, NY, a major residential drug-free therapeutic community. Brooklyn College of the City University of New York (CUNY) is the collaborating academic institution. Since its inception more than 300 student/residents have earned 4,000 matriculated credits with an overall B-average.

The Daytop Miniversity has developed a successful model of matriculated college level education in residental drug-free treatment. Its students have successfully continued in their pursuits of higher education.

The authors wish to acknowledge the assistance given this Project and its staff by Ms. Lisa Pepe.

They have earned — since the start of the project — and continue to earn undergraduate and graduate degrees in the Physical Sciences (Physics); Social Sciences (Human Development; Sociological Research) and Humanities. It has provided new opportunities for high risk clients. It has empirically demonstrated that it can facilitate and intensify the treatment/rehabilitation experience. An empirical data base is being generated from a rigorous investigation of this Project. Such a unique body of information has the potential to provide new findings which will improve the treatment process and the significant development of human potential.

Although grant support for the acedemic component terminated in early 1982, the Project has expanded its scope beyond college level programming. It now includes a range of technical training programs and pre-college programs for residents. Programs to support professional training for staff development have also been instituted.

The foundation, organization and administration of the eligible Daytop residents who have earned matriculated credits from Brooklyn College of the City University of New York is the history of this Project and is chronicled elsewhere — **Daytop Miniversity: College Training Within a Therapeutic Community**.

This chapter describes one aspect of the major quantitative evaluation results relative to the Miniversity as a program enhancement for drug-free residential TC treatment. It focuses on the empirical assessment of the development of self esteem and self concept among addict/abusers.

Miniversity Research Evaluation Overview

The Daytop Miniversity Project 1979-1984 is the first documented successful deployment of a treatment intervention research experiment in a major drug-free TC setting. As such Phase 2 of the Project employed an Experimental Group (N = 110) which included subjects' participation in both Miniversity and TC treatment or assignment to a Control Group (N = 59) which was involvement in the TC treatment track only.

Thus the Miniversity's Research Evaluation incorporated several robust research design characteristics which strengthen the findings and their applicability. These features included random assignment of subjects, use of Experimental and Control Groups and a longitudinal repeated measures paradigm. Repeated measures were obtained for both the Experimental and Control Groups.

Additional features should be noted in regard to the quality of this unique experimental project. Pre-tests were given to all potential subjects prior to random assignment to either experimental or control conditions. Thus there was no selection bias based upon measurement of the self concept dependent variables. Means of the Experimental and Control Groups do not differ significantly from each other on these dimensions.

The successful deployment of a randomly assigned paradigm in the Phase 2 study was accomplished after a previous Demonstration-Evaluation Phase 1 (1979-1980) 18 month Miniversity deployment. The Phase 1 Miniversity utilized a carefully matched Control Group — matched identically by group means on 21 critical variables. These variables included demographic, drug history, social, educational history and scores on intelligence and self concept measures. While these subjects were all qualified to Miniversity students the matched Controls self-selected not to participate in this combined education/treatment project.

Academic Completion

The enhancement effect of the Miniversity was evident in influencing a notable course completion rate. In a per semester analysis initial results indicate that of those resident/students who began Semester 1 and Semester 2, 88.5 percent completed the required course work and earned matriculated final grades. These semesters occurred contemporaneous with months 3 thru 14 of the residential treatment program.

Semester 3, which occurs in the downstate NYC Reentry phase — months 14-18, had a course completion rate of 70 percent.

An analysis of completion rates for the total three semester Miniversity track which spans a twelve month time period indicates that approximately 50 percent of those residents who begin Semester 1 continue successfully to earn final grades at the end of Semester 3.

These rates compare favorably with completion rates for post-secondary college level participation with students in traditional non-rehabilitation campus settings.

Scholastic/Academic Achievement

Resident/students who participated in matriculated Miniversity course work have provided a reliable measure of areas of academic strengths that may be used for future program development efforts outside of the college-Miniversity proper. Analyses of grade achievement (earned grades) were conducted in the areas of English, Mathematics, Computer Sciences, Behavioral Sciences, Health, Geology and Speech. Earned course grades in each of these areas were subjected to quantitative analyses. The earned mean grade point average is based on a 4.00 Grade Point Average (G.P.A.) where 4.00 is equivalent to a college level of "A" grade.

Analysis of earned Grade Point Average in each academic area revealed that the resident/students earned a "B" average in Computer Science and "Bffl" grade average in Human Sexuality and Human Physiology. Grades earned in English, Speech and Behavioral Sciences which included courses in Psychology, Economics, Political Science and Education ranged from a "C⅔" to a "Bffl" average.

The positive performance in the quantitative areas of **Computer Science** and **Mathematics** is noteworthy and highlights the training and future occupational potential of the Miniversity participants. It particularly emphasizes that there is untapped intellectual potential among individuals in drug-free TC treatment and rehabilitation.

Slightly lower but positive grade averages in the other subjects, particularly English and Behavioral Science, is seeming a result of a reduced fund of general information. These conclusions are based on repeated student-classroom observation and faculty feedback to the Evaluation Team. Many individuals, for example, rarely, if ever, read books, newspapers, or watched informational television during their years of addiction or abuse, and if they did their attention and retention ability was notably impaired or diminished.

The notable results reflected in these data have been applied in a two year planning process at Daytop Village and are currently supporting the design of a new program for technical training in Word Processing and Microcomputer Operations. This is one example of the expanded scope of the Miniversity concept for TC residential treatment.

Beta II Intelligence
Measure of Non-Verbal Ability and Achievement

The Revised Beta II was used as a measure of general intellectual ability. It is non-verbal measure which yields an estimate of ability which can be expressed as an I.Q. The average Beta I.Q. for the Miniversity Group and the Control Group was 95.5, equivalent to an average level intelligence classification.

Initial regression analyses using full Beta I.Q. and subtest scores for the six subtests yielded no statistically significant relationships between the dependent variables of Completion of Treatment or Grade Point Average for the Miniversity Group.

The findings indicate that despite the rigors of residential TC treatment, a cohort of drug-free addict/abusers with an Average level Non-Verbal I.Q. estimate, have achieved greater than average levels of cognitive competency and enhanced self esteem. The unique Miniversity within TC environment provides for a new opportunity for social and academic learning. From what has been developed, the successful TC can now offer a new model and challenge to formal education systems in the intellectual and emotional development of troubled young adults.

Project Research Evaluation Design

The Project's evaluation/research question concerns whether an effect of Miniversity can be discerned over and above any effect of the ordinary Daytop treatment. Although decreased use of controlled substances would seem a logical outcome upon which to evaluate treatment efforts, it would not serve within a resedental drug-free environment, as here. Instead the components of self concept, including self esteem and self perceived pathology were used as an index of the Daytop TC Program's ability to improve the emotional health of residents and clients. Theory and research indicating depleted self esteem among substance abusers as well as considerations in the psychopathology of addiction guided the choice. The components of self esteem were quantified operationally by the subscales of the Tennessee Self Concept Scale (TSCS). Thus, this aspect of the evaluation research question specifically concerns gains on the subscales of the TSCS; over time for all Daytop participants; and in an enhanced fashion (either sooner or of greater magnitude) for the Daytop residents assigned to Miniversity.

Self Concept as a Criterion for Rehabilitation Planning and Progress

The developer of the TSCS stated that:

> In rehabilitation the client's self concept should serve as a helpful criterion in two ways. First, it should assist in the determination of final objectives which are appropriate and also in the initial decision of where and how rehabilitation should begin. The evidence indicates that individuals with

highly negative and deviant self concepts are high risks for continuation and satisfactory performance in any activities. In many instances some kind of "self concept habilitation" may be needed before vocational or other phases of rehabilitation should be attempted.

TSCS Assessment Schedule

Resident/students where assigned to Experimental or Control Group completely at random from among the pool of college qualified individuals. Non-college qualified are not included in any aspect of the study. Groups have unequal n by experimenter's choice, that is, the unequal n do not represent a feature of the data but rather express the experimenter's intent to provide augmented service for as many individuals as possible while retaining an adequately sized Control Group for research purposes. Measurements were taken at intervals approximately the length of an university semester, with the first testing occurring after at least 90 to 180 days in Daytop TC treatment and before the beginning of Miniversity courses for those assigned to that condition. The final testing was scheduled after all course completion and prior to completion from the Daytop Reentry program.

Variables/Analyses

The 29 subscales of the TSCS were designated as the dependent variables for analysis. These operationalize changes in self perception indexing gains attributable to the treatment and augmented Miniversity treatment process. The independent or grouping variable was membership in Experimental or Control Group, where The Experimental group received Miniversity courses in addition to ordinary Daytop treatment and Control Group received ordinary Daytop treatment alone.

On the 29 subscales of the TSCS, the Total Positive Scale summarizes the 8 main scales measuring separate dimensions of the self concept. Figure 1 displays the Total Positive Self Concept scores for the Miniversity and Control Groups. The data collection occurred over the Project's 30 month study period and represents four points in treatment — Repetition 1 = 6 months; Repetition 2 = 10 months; Repetition 3 = 14 months; Repetition 4 = 18 months.

The results reveal an orderly and significant progression of self concept for both groups between testing on Repetition 2 thru Repetition 4 reflecting months 6 thru 18 of TC treatment. They particularly highlight the treatment enhancement of the Miniversity by demonstrating

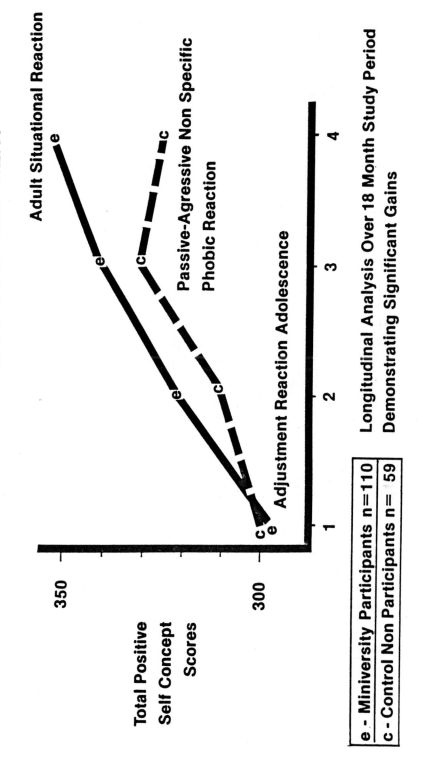

DISPLAY OF SELF CONCEPT DEVELOPMENT

Total Positive Self Concept Scores

Longitudinal Analysis Over 18 Month Study Period
Demonstrating Significant Gains

e - Miniversity Participants n=110
c - Control Non Participants n= 59

greater acceleration and magnitude of change. The Control Group achieves gains at a slower rate than the Experimental Group. They also differ in absolute levels with regard to specific aspects of self esteem and self concept. As such the Control Group members may require extended TC treatment exposure to achieve a more integrated and positive level of self concept. These issues are the focus of analyses of longer term outcomes.

Empirical Verification of the Daytop TC Treatment Process and Miniversity Enhancement

The results in Figure 1 are also relevant to the study of the process of TC treatment. Previous TC literature has produced results indicating a relationship between TC treatment and the reduction of pathological levels of anxiety and depression. Several studies have reported reductions in general levels of generic psychopathology and maladjustment as a result of TC treatment. The current Miniversity results have found support for these trends. It has moreover uncovered the kind of self concept and psychological growth that is part of successful TC treatment and as such is helping to formulate empirically based clinical criteria.

Figure 1 is a clear depiction of the above in that it reflects the pattern of total self concept development in Daytop TC treatment. The Miniversity and Control Groups appear similar to populations classified as "Adjustment Reaction to Adolescence" at Repetition 1 or at Pre test. Both groups progress in a positive and consistent manner with the Miniversity group making significantly greater gains sooner by Repetition 2. At Repetition 3 (14 months in treatment) no statistically significant difference exists between the groups. It appears that the Control Group during this period has kept clinical pace with the Miniversity group. At Repetition 4 (18 months — Reentry Phase) the Miniversity is again significantly different from the Control Group. Moreover, Miniversity completers have achieved self esteem scores which are more age-appropriate and comparable with the "Adult Situation Reaction." Members of the Control Group have also achieved adult-like scores but share a configuration with persons classified as "Phobic Reactions" or "Non-Specific Passive Aggressive Personalities" — suggesting that individual clinical interventions may be constructive for these individuals.

The importance of the above findings is that they specifically support the developmental clinical framework of the TC philosophy. This is a clinical approach which assumes that rehabilitation requires not only reduction of psychopathology or maladjustment but necessitates a concommitant development of self concept and self esteem. It assumes that to characterize addicts and abusers who seek TC treatment as sociopathic, deviant or distinct type of abusers minimizes more substantive issues related to personality and lifestyle approaches. TC treatment philosophy emphasizes that the addiction and abuse is an immature, inappropriate, at times childlike avoidance response to conflict resolution. Thus, what these data reflect unequivocally is that participation in TC treatment can enhance the development of self concept and self esteem. An even greater self esteem enhancement and benefit now exists for individuals who participate in TC treatment and structured academic training.

Ongoing research and evaluation efforts at Daytop Village's Department of Research and Development are continuing to define more specific components of the self concept construct that are both necessary and sufficient for clinical success.

Miniversity's Positive Influence in Increasing Retention in TC Treatment

The Miniversity has been virtually a landmark study in providing the first documented intervention to positively influence the retention of residents in TC treatment. While analytical work in progress is highlighting differences among residents who leave treatment in contrast to those who complete treatment, the effect of the Miniversity is unequivocal.

About 15 percent fewer of the Miniversity Group drop out of TC treatment during the first 12 months, compared to 30 percent from the randomly assigned Control Group. This finding, although not statistically significant, is particularly notable because previous research at Daytop and other TCs suggest that length of participation in program is related to a more positive post program adjustment. Also the first year of treatment is particularly critical in influencing both psychological and social change while it is also the period when most residents leave treatment against program advice. These data thus suggest that providing a structural educational/training track within the TC treatment environment is likely to increase the retention rate for particular residents. A comparison with the self concept data also indicates that it is within the first two semesters that the most dramatic and significant gains are effected and achieved.

A further examination of the data reveals that the pattern of an improved retention rate for the first 12 months of treatment for the Miniversity Group reverses in the months 13-24 or the second year of treatment. Retention rates for the Miniversity and Control Groups are virtually equivalent for the past 24 month period of treatment.

Structured clinically documented observations and carefully measured self concept gains suggest that such a program has a direct positive impact on self concept development and in turn positively influences retention during the more critical TC treatment phase. During the second year of treatment many of the Miniversity students seem to be even more prepared to return to the general community and choose not to participate in a scheduled and supervised reentry phase.

Comment

The Daytop Miniversity is a major programmatic and scientific effort designed to enhance the Therapeutic Community field. The Project continues to generate new empirical information about the TC as a contemporary treatment environment for the rehabilitation of addicts and substance abusers; for facilitating behavior change; for enhancing the development of mental health and for providing college education for non-traditional students. Its outcomes have reaffirmed the untapped intellectual potential of persons who have been addicts or severe substance abusers. Moreover, it has developed a new model which integrates both academic and social learning as a synergistic therapeutic experience. The rigorous research and evaluation of the Project continues to suggest strategies by which to explore the process of critical therapeutic change within the TC. A recently completed long-term follow-up study using self concept and social adjustment data base is building the foundation for measuring "self efficacy" with this unique clinical population. In an era when addiction and substance abuse are such prominent international socio-psychological issues, the outcomes of the Project are helping to refine the scope and impact of effective TC treatment.

CHAPTER 11

CLIENT EVALUATIONS OF THERAPEUTIC COMMUNITIES AND RETENTION

WARD S. CONDELLI

L ITTLE COMPREHENSIVE research has been done on how clients in therapeutic communities for drug addicts evaluate these programs and its treatment process. How clients evaluate their programs is likely to effect how long they stay there, how much they benefit from treatment, and the extent to which they have successful outcomes after they leave the program. Client evaluations of the treatment process of therapeutic communities could be useful for improving its effectiveness and increasing retention and favorable outcomes. Length of stay has been reported to be the most important factor in successful outcomes from therapeutic communities (De Leon, 1983; 1984a).

Many evaluations of therapeutic communities and other drug treatment programs have concentrated on assessing how differences in the backgrounds and characteristics of clients effect retention. The domains investigated include: sociodemographic variables; family and early background characteristics; social and psychological assessments; schooling and employment; leisure activities and peer relationships; history of criminal activity and involvement with the legal system; type, frequency, extent and patterns of drug use; and motivations for joining the program. These domains have been fairly well investigated and the results show that they do not explain much variance in retention (De Leon, 1984b).

Research on the role of external pressure in retention in therapeutic communities has viewed contradictory findings. For example, one study found that the relationship between these variables was positive (Aron &

Daily, 1976), three studies found that it was negative (Biase, 1974; Nash, Waldorf, Foster & Kyllingstadt, 1974; Waldorf, 1973), and one study found that it was of no significance (Joe & Simpson, 1976). These contradictory findings may have been due to differences between samples of clients in terms of how long they had been in the program, some studies not clearly identifying what pressure was applied by the legal system on clients to join the program, and other studies not taking into account pressure from the client's significant others. More recent research found that the relationship between legal pressure and retention was positive and strongest for newer clients to the program, and that clients stayed longer in the program when they reported pressure from significant others (Condelli, 1980).

Research that has taken into account only external pressure and differences in the backgrounds and characteristics of clients has left a lot of unexplained variance in retention. This suggests that the predictive value of other variables needs to be investigated. Two domains of variables that have been overlooked by all of these studies are client evaluations of their programs and its treatment process. The objective of the present research was to analyze the relationship between these variables and retention.

Method

A 25-page questionnaire was administered to 139 clients in five residential drug treatment programs in New Jersey in 1978. This sample of clients was about half of the populations in these programs that were eligible (i.e, 18 years of age or older) to participate in the research. The programs included two traditional therapeutic communities, two nontraditional therapeutic communities, and one work program. The questionnaire took into account client background variables and external pressure to join the program. In addition, clients were asked about how much they needed the program and the sacrifices required to stay there, the behavior expected by the program, how important it was to staff and clients that they stay in the program, and their overall evaluations of the program.

External Pressure

Indices were constructed to represent two kinds of external pressure on clients to join the program. These were: (1) the number of months of jail clients estimated that they faced if they left the program before graduation; and (2) the degree of pressure that clients said was exerted on them by significant others to join the program. The significant others included family members and spouses or lovers. The number of months of jail faced by clients were recoded into four categories for the legal pressure variable. These ranged from zero (no pressure) to three (clients faced with the most number of months of jail). For the significant others' pressure variable, clients were assigned to one of three categories on the basis of the significant other who exerted the greatest amount of pressure on the client to join the program. The categories ranged from zero (no pressure) to two (high pressure), with the middle category representing clients with low pressure from significant others.

A cross tabulation of the legal and significant others' pressure variables revealed that only 16 or the 139 clients came to the program without any external pressure. Twenty-two of the clients entered the program with legal pressure and no pressure from significant others, and 31 clients joined with pressure from significant others and no legal pressure. About half of the clients joined the program with both types of pressure. Thus, external pressure appeared to be an important inducement for these clients to join their programs.

Needs and Sacrifice

Clients were asked how much they needed the program, and how much sacrifice it required to stay there. Responses to these questions were coded on six-point Likert-scales. About one-third of the clients indicated very much need for the program, and two-thirds said they needed it much or very much. Forty-five percent of the clients felt it required very much sacrifice to stay in the program, and over three-quarters felt that staying in the program required much sacrifice. Responses to both questions were recoded into a three-point scale that ranged from very much need or sacrifice to less than much need or sacrifice.

Clients were also asked to specify how many months they needed to be a resident at their program. The mean and modal responses were, respectively, 10 and 12 months. Responses to this question were recoded into three categories of nearly equal size. These were: zero to six months; seven to eleven months; and more than eleven months.

Behavior Expected by Program

Clients were asked questions about the behavior that was expected by their programs. One question was: "To what extent is conforming to the behavior expected here an important part of the program, or to what extent is this behavior stupid?" Nearly two-thirds of the clients thought that the behavior was an important part of the program, and only three indicated that it was stupid. The others scored the behavior between these two poles or said they did not know whether it was important or stupid. Responses to this question were recoded into two categories: clients who indicated that the behavior was important; and clients who indicated otherwise.

Another question asked of clients was: "How hard is it for you to conform to the behavior expected by the program?" Fifty-six of the clients responded that it was very hard or hard to conform to this behavior, and the remainder felt that it was less than hard. Responses to this question were recoded into these two categories.

Staff and Residents

Clients were asked how important it was to staff and residents that they stay in the program. Forty percent indicated that it was very important or important to staff that they stay, 31% said it was of medium importance, and the rest felt that their staying was less than of medium importance of staff. The question which asked clients how important it was to residents that they stay in the program had a similar distribution of responses. Thus, responses to both questions were recoded into three categories: very important or important; medium importance; and less than medium importance.

Global Program Evaluations

Global evaluations of the program were measured with a 80-item comparative evaluation scale that had a format which was similar to the semantic differential (Cf. Bredemeier, 1978; 1979; Condelli, 1980). The scale asked clients to evaluate their programs and high school on multiple dimensions. The clients were asked to evaluate high school because it provided a common institutional reference point from which to compare their evaluations of the program. In order to make this comparison, evaluation scores of the program were divided by evaluation scores of high school for each item on the comparative evaluation scale. An analysis of these scores revealed that clients tended to evaluate their programs in roughly equal frequencies either better than, the same as, or worse than high school on most of the scores. The comparative evaluation scale scores were then recoded into these three categories and factor analyzed. This indicated that there were six factors which were significant in terms of the amount of common variance they explained and theoretically congruent with what the respective dimensions purported to measure. Composite scores were output for each of the items in the factor analysis and high positive scores indicated favorable evaluations of the program.

Length of Stay

Two variables were used for measures of length of stay in the program. These were: (1) the number of days clients spent in the program prior to the administration of the questionnaires; and (2) the number of days clients stayed at the program 100 days after taking the questionnaire. An analysis indicated that there was significant interaction between these two variables and that the second measure was influenced by the first one (Cf. De Leon & Schwartz, 1984c). Consequently, these two measures of length of stay were added together and divided by 30, producing the number of months clients spent at the program 100 days after the administration of the questionnaire. The main length of stay for this measure was 7.1 months, with a standard deviation of 3.7 months. The mean and modal lengths of stay were, respectively, 5.0 and 6.8 months.

Path Analysis

This research used path analysis to explore the relationship between the variables in this study. This involved computing a series of hierarchical regression equations to test whether variables that were posited to effect other variables did so significantly. A general F Test, referred to as "Model I Error," was used to test the significance of the incremental increases in the variance explained by independent variables as they were brought into the equation (Cf. Cohen & Cohen, 1975). Hierarchical regression analysis was used to partial out variance explained by variables brought into the equation in preceeding steps. Variables were excluded from the analysis when it was found that they did not directly or indirectly effect length of stay in the program.

Results

Figure 1 shows a model which depicts the results of the path analysis for this study. Seven variables were found to directly effect length of stay in the program. These variables, and the percentage of unique variance in length of stay that they explained, were: (1) client's age (.04); (2) legal pressure (.04); (3) significant others' pressure (.02); (4) a comparison of the traditional therapeutic communities with the work program (.05); (5) client rating of the program on the salience dimension on the comparative evaluation scale (.04); (6) the number of months that clients felt they needed to be a resident at their program (.07); and (7) how important clients thought it was to staff that they stay in the program (.06). The seven variables accounted for 32% of the variance in length of stay in the program.

Figure 1 shows the interrelationships between these variables. Starting with the age of clients, and moving from left to right on the path model, the following may be inferred about how the variables effected one another. Older clients were more likely than younger clients to enter the program with legal pressure, report no pressure from significant others to join the program, reside at the work program rather than at one of the non-traditional therapeutic communities, and to stay in the program for fewer months.

Clients who joined the program with legal pressure were more likely than clients who joined the program without this pressure to enter the program with high pressure from significant others, feel that they needed to be a resident at their programs for many months, and to stay longer at the program. Clients who joined the program with high pressure from significant others stayed there more months than clients who joined without this pressure.

The next variables in the path model are comparisons between the two types of therapeutic communities and the work program. The model indicates that clients in the traditional therapeutic communities rated their programs lower on the salience dimension on the comparative evaluation scale and stayed at their programs for a shorter amount of the time than clients at the work program. Compared with clients in the work program, those in the non-traditional therapeutic communities thought it was more important to staff that they stay in program.

The last set of variables in the path model are client evaluations of their programs and its treatment process. The model shows that clients who stayed longest in the program felt they needed to be a resident there for many months, rated their programs high on the salience dimension on the comparative evaluation scale, and said it was important to staff that they stay in the program.

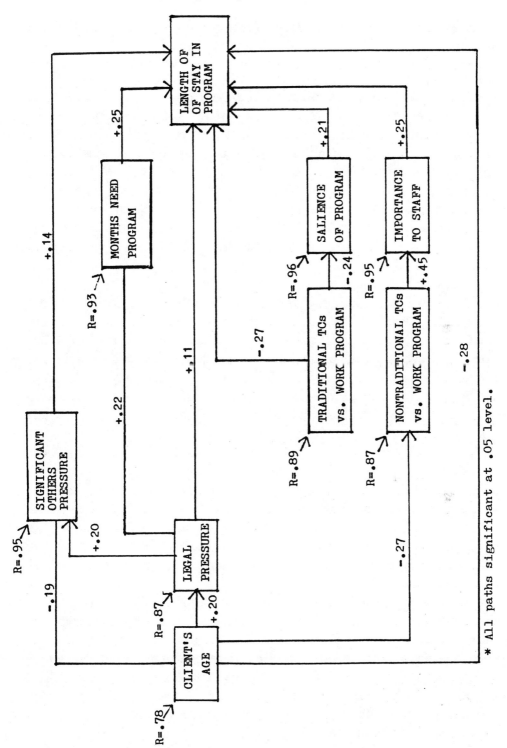

* All paths significant at .05 level.

Discussion

The sample for this study was a cross-section of clients in five residential programs for drug addicts. While this sample consisted of approximately half of the populations at these programs that were eligible (i.e., 18 years of age or older) to participate in the research, it is not known whether it was representative of those populations. The research design leaves it unclear whether some of the findings may be due to selective dropout, or to changes in clients resulting from the time they spent in the program prior to the administration of the questionnaire. Cross-sectional research designs have an inherent problem of questionable internal validity (Campbell & Stanley, 1963; Labouvie, 1976). Consequently, the findings of this exploratory study should be regarded as tentative until they can be confirmed or disconfirmed by studies with better research designs.

This research found a significant positive relationship between legal pressure and length of stay in the program. An analysis was done of how the four conditions of the legal pressure variable were related to retention. This revealed that, while the relationship held across the conditions of this variable, there were minor differences between the retention rates of clients who reported low, medium, and high legal pressure. Thus, what appears to affect retention most is not how much pressure is applied by the legal system, but whether or not there is legal pressure.

The path analysis for this study indicated that both legal and significant others' pressure were intervening variables between the client's age and length of stay in the program. Age was found to be positively related to legal pressure and negatively related to pressure from significant others. Legal pressure indirectly affected retention through significant others' pressure. This suggests that legal pressure tends to activate significant others to exert pressure on younger clients to join the program to avoid prison.

In the past, therapeutic communities have had ambivalent relationships with the significant others of clients. On one hand these programs have encouraged significant others to become more involved with clients. This was in part done to discourage significant others from disrupting the client's treatment and pulling clients out of the program. On the other hand, therapeutic communities have regarded the client's significant others as agents which encourage and reinforce drug addiction (Yablonsky, 1970). In contrast, many of the clients in this research reported that significant others applied pressure on them to join the program, and that is important to their significant others that they stay in the program. Moreover, significant others' pressure was found to be positively related to length of stay in the program. These findings indicate that therapeutic communities may increase retention rates by finding ways for significant others to encourage clients to stay in the program and take a more active role in the client's treatment.

Clients who stayed longest in the program were those who were residents at programs other than the traditional therapeutic communities, who rated their programs high on the salience dimension on the comparative evaluation scale, and who said it was important to staff that they stay in the program. Clients in the traditional therapeutic communities rated their programs lower on the salience dimension than those in the work program. Compared to clients in the non-traditional therapeutic communities, those in the work program said it was less important to staff that they stay in the program. These findings suggest that the traditional therapeutic communities in this study could increase retention rates were they to find ways to make their programs more salient to clients. Alternatively, the work program in this study could reduce attrition by encouraging its staff to demonstrate that it was important that clients stay in the program.

Length of stay in the program was found to be positively related to the number of months that clients felt they needed to be a resident at their program. Most of the clients in this study thought they needed to stay at their programs for somewhat fewer months than are usually required by these programs. These findings imply that retention rates could be increased by having the staff at these programs explain more thoroughly to clients the rationale for the length of the treatment program. It is also possible that these programs need to consider shortening their treatment phases and perhaps lengthening their re-entry phases to reduce client attrition.

This study found that client evaluations of their programs and its treatment process accounted for far more variance in retention than did the background variables of clients. Moreover, most of the variance in length of stay that was explained by the background variables was due to legal and significant others' pressure. This suggests that the variables over which therapeutic communities have the greatest control are those which have the most influence on retention. More research is needed to understand how programs could be modified to improve the effectiveness of treatment and reduce client attrition. Clients would be one good source of information for evaluating those modifications.

CHAPTER 12

SIDE BETS AND SECONDARY ADJUSTMENTS IN THERAPEUTIC COMMUNITIES

J. DAVID HAWKINS
NORMAN WACKER

INTRODUCTION

G OFFMAN has described both the encompassing character of total institutions (1961:6) and the ubiquitous presence of collectively sustained secondary adjustments among residents in them (1961:199). Secondary adjustments are practices which do not directly challenge the staff of a total institution, but allow residents to obtain forbidden satisfactions or obtain permitted ones by forbidden means. Goffman notes, "Secondary adjustments demonstrate to the practitioner that he has some selfhood and personal autonomy beyond the grasp of the organization" (1961:314). He sees secondary adjustments as reactions **against** the strains put on self by the encompassing character of total institutions.

In this paper, we suggest that residents in total institutions may engage in secondary adjustments not only because they are rebelling against encompassing controls, but because they see their stay in these institutions as temporary. We suggest that total institutions are not successful in eliminating reference to perspectives beyond the institution because they are not total in the temporal sense. In most total institutions, residents know they will ultimately return to the outside world, hence the concept of "short time" in prisons. From this perspective, secondary adjustments may reflect residents' **commitments to** the perspectives of the world from which they have come and to which they will return, rather than **rebellion against** the institution in which they find themselves.

Method

This perspective emerged from study of one total institution, a therapeutic community (TC) established for the treatment of drug abusers. One of the authors spent four weeks as a participant observer in an urban TC with a population of 20 residents. The observer was identified as a researcher to other residents, but otherwise participated in the TC as a member governed by the same rules and regulations as other TC residents with two exceptions. The observer was allowed to write field notes during a specified period each day and the observer left the TC once a week to meet with the other author. These discussions were recorded and transcribed. Importantly, the orientation of other residents toward the observer was as veterans to a naive newcomer. As more advanced members of a self-help program, they had an institutional responsibility to educate the initiate, and residents shared with the observer accounts of their own initiation to the TC, as well as the skills necessary for getting along in the TC.

Research Setting

TCs share a treatment philosophy about the nature and sources of drug addiction and the pathways to the user's cure. TC treatment philosophy assumes the user has never reached a mature state of psychic development and withdraws from the conflicts of emotional life into drug-induced euphorias, false personal imageries, and the inhumane social codes of the drug culture (Washburne et al., 1977:17). TC therapy attempts to remove the user from association with his prior social network, to strip him of the self-images and values of the drug subculture, and to socialize him to the behaviors and values of conventional life. The treatment goals of TCs are broad, seeking to effect comprehensive personality and behavior change (Catalano et al., 1983).

This comprehensive resocialization process requires the resident's development of a new self-image by participation in an intensive self-help process. Frequent group therapy and encounter sessions, daily seminars in TC self-help concepts, strict rules restricting all interactions between clients to program models, and an "argot" dictated by the TC are means by which the therapeutic philosophy is operationalized. Clients are in residence 24 hours a day. Because TCs attempt to supplant the home world of the resident and to reorient him to identification with an alternative to his native milieu, they have many of the attributes of total institutions.

In the literature, TC resocialization of clients has been described as so intensive and encompassing that clients have no latitude to act in ways not allowed by the TC code without experiencing negative sanctions (Hawkins, & Wacker, 1983; Johnson, 1976; Washburn, 1977). The literature does not discuss collectively sustained secondary adjustments. This research report indicates that such adjustments occur in at least some TCs.

Institutional Mechanisms for Resocialization

The major task of TCs, as of all total institutions, is to remove residents from identification with and use of the perspectives of previous reference groups, and to encourage residents to adopt the perspective of the institution (Goffman, 1961:6-60). TCs attempt to strip the self by forcing residents to focus on the "here and now" of the TC and by blocking reference to past identities and norms of other reference groups. Residents are prohibited contact with outsiders during the first several weeks or months of residence and certain topics of conversation are prohibited; e.g., past life, religion, politics, criminal activity, drugs, and sex. In order to move about the TC without constant accompaniment of another resident, initiates must memorize and repeat the prohibited list to a senior resident.

One of the central mechanisms used for generating behavior and identity change during this initial phase is the "pullup." The pullup is one process for restructuring the self-identities of residents. A pullup in a sharp verbal command shouted at the offender by another resident. The phrase shouted is "get a grip." In every case, the offender must respond with the words "thank you," spoken in a calm voice without emotion. Any response which implies emotion or irritation is characterized as reacting and is strictly forbidden. Any resident observing the following situations is required to use the pullup:

1. Any lapse in awareness of personal property or tools, including dropping or spilling anything, leaving any tools or personal property, such as a coffee cup, unattended for any period, however brief.
2. Failure to complete any household responsibility to perfection. (Rigorous inspections of all task assignments are routine.)
3. Displaying a negative attitude either in responding to a verbal command or pullup, or any instance of moodiness, anger, or depression in interactions between residents outside a group sessions.

4. Talking about any forbidden topics: sex, religion, politics, drugs, crime, or one's deviant past outside of group therapy sessions.
5. Displaying negative feelings about the program or other residents outside of group sessions.

Receiving two or more pullups for the same behavior may be considered repeated behavior and can enmesh the resident in more rigorous and aversive program sanctions, such as "trims" (intense verbal confrontations mounted by three group members to which the resident is not permitted to respond) or "learning experiences" (cumbersome cardboard signs worn about the neck, lifejackets, haircuts, or indefinite assignment to maintenance details over and above the normal work duties).

Residents encountering pullups during their first days in the TC witness a reversal of the social codes they have lived by on the streets. In the TC, monitoring the behavior of peers, calling the behavior to the attention of the offending resident with a pullup, and in the case of more serious infractions, bringing behavior to the attention of the group coordinator, is referred to as help. This system of mutual surveillance violates the norms of the drug culture against "snitching." The system of pullups and "bringing behavior" makes residents increasingly aware of the conflict between the expectations of the street and the expectations of the TC.

Residents frequently described the conflict they faced as initiates when first confronted with pullups. One resident testified to the pressure the system put on her personal code of ethics. She claimed that other women attempted to evade this pressure by never bringing behavior to the attention of the coordinator. She said that she knew that if any of the behavior among the "sisters" was to be "brought," she would have to bring it. She said this role made her feel like a spy.

Residents admitted that they often avoided giving pullups because it made them feel uncomfortable and foolish. One resident who had received a learning experience (a large cardboard sign worn around the neck) for not using a pullup during an altercation with another resident, was asked to speak on the topic of giving help in an impromptu seminar. The resident recounted that as an ex-convict who had lived by the rules of the street and penitentiary for many years, he had thought of pullups and bringing behavior as violating confidences. He said he had seen using the self-help tools as hostile acts toward other residents. Later, during a public testimonial in a group therapy session, he stated that he now realized that use of the pullup was a way of showing care and concern for fellow residents, and that using the pullup was "all about help."

Nevertheless, this same resident told the observer in private conversation that he was not about to bring anyone's behavior to public scrutiny if he did not have to. Similarly, in three instances, residents confessed after bringing someone's behavior up in the group that they had not used pullups at the time of the alleged incidents.

Residents reluctant to accept their responsibility to give pullups could be confronted in group sessions and stigmatized as uncaring and neglectful of the needs of other residents. In eight group sessions, the observer witnessed 13 incidents in which residents were subjected to sustained verbal confrontation by staff and other residents upon their motives and their characters for not using pullup. In two instances, these verbal assaults were followed by learning experiences requiring the offending resident to wear a large cardboard sign which characterized the resident as "unaware," "hurtful," and "uncaring." Two residents who had failed to confront another resident in a group therapy session were subjected to a family trim (a systematic and sustained verbal confrontation mounted to each member of the family in succession). In such ways, residents seeking to avoid implication in TC treatment were drawn into increasingly dramatic displays of the power of the TC to stigmatize perspectives held over from the prior life.

Pullups also functioned to draw residents' attention to the present and away from casual reference to the larger society. Residents found that events of no consequence outside the TC became charged with consequence in the TC. Residents could be pulled up for an improperly made bed, a moment of inattention during group or seminar, leaving a residue of disinfectant in a shower stall, dropping a piece of silverware, or leaving a cigarette unattended in an ashtray. The lapse was broadcast to everyone within earshot of the pullup. Thus the execution of the most mundane tasks could be tied to the resident's image in the eyes of the group with an attendant impact on his or her self-esteem. For some residents, self-esteem and personal status become implicated in TC norms and the in-house status structure. One resident repeatedly advertised the fact, with pride, that he had cleaned the stove 11 times in a row without receiving a pullup. Another resident, when asked by the observer to explain the logic behind pullups, talked at length of the connection between pullups and a resident's sense of self, as well as the impact of pullups on the group's perception of the resident:

> You've got to understand that junkies are people who live their lives by doing things halfway and saying "that's good enough for me," but doing a halfway job isn't good enough when there is a man paying the bills. Lots of dope

fiends lose jobs by dropping things and leaving tools funky and shuffling along like they generally don't give a damn. The thing here with the pullup is there is always someone watching you every minute, telling you how what you are doing is coming off to them. No one wants to look a fool, so if you are aware that what you are doing is looking like a fool, you want to put a stop to it. It makes you get on top of things so you don't need getting pulled up for not making your bed, so everyone knows you keep a funky room and maybe start thinking you do other things funky, too.

Residents who felt that seemingly trivial incidents could diminish their prestige in the eyes of other residents intensified their focus on the minuteness of TC living so as to avoid humiliating characterizations of self by other residents. In this way, they moved closer to identifying the TC group as the critical reference group in which their self-concept was to be secured.

War Stories as Secondary Adjustments

We have described an encompassing set of institutional mechanisms of resocialization which are powerful agents for effecting a conversion to new values and modes of behavior. However, in the TC, these mechanisms were not wholly successful in separating residents from identification with and reference to the drug subculture. Perhaps the clearest example of this is the fact that residents in this TC continued to share "war stories" of the streets with each other, recounting their drug experiences in private times and spaces they created for themselves in the TC. Residents engaged in these secondary adjustments in spite of the fact that they were clearly forbidden and risked severe punishments. Even clients who were otherwise engaged in use of the TCs self-help tools and exhibited high incidence of compliant behaviors, often privately shared "war stories" of their exploits on the streets.

One client spoke to the observer at length of the strategies he used on the street to recruit women for prostitution. The client described in detail his mastery of manipulative body language which he used as a tool to maneuver his mark into an attitude of receptivity to his proposal. He boasted that he could always tell when a women was receptive and would not rebuff his approach. He also spoke with pride of having grown up as a child on the streets and having heightened powers of observation which allowed him to spot shortchange artists, pickpockets, ripoffs, and potential violent incidents in an instant. This information was volunteered privately. This resident did not appear to be rebelling against TC life. He spoke frequently of the desire to advance in the TC status structure, and of his commitment to his personal rehabilitation. He expressed a desire to learn the techniques of TC therapy so that he could "really do something after I've gotten myself together in here." In group, he described the realization that his life as a pimp had not been a life of mastery at all, adding "and then when I woke up one morning and the women were all gone, I was a sad case, I didn't have no hustle. It hit me that I wasn't keeping them, they was keeping me."

Another resident described a period of trouble-free addiction lasting several months. She had amassed a sizable amount of money; she had the use of a luxury home with a swimming pool; and she had secured a trustworthy connection and a stable supply of high-quality heroin. The resident described idyllic summer days spent at poolside lost in the euphoria of sunshine, easy living, and her heroin-induced high. After recounting this story, she added a disclaimer. Her voice sounded a scornful note of self-judgment as she invoked the TC image of drug addicts as if to censor what had gone before: "kicked back . . . typical dope fiend . . . anything to kick back, a real junkie's holiday."

Another resident who was high in the TC structure of self-help responsibility, who manifested a high degree of involvement in TC processes, and who spoke frequently of wanting to found his own TC, also told the observer of "an incredible feeling of love" surrounding his activities as a major dealer of cocaine.

TC residents invested large amounts of time and personal resources in the procurement and use of heroin prior to entry into the TC. Street life can be dangerous and competitive but rewarding as well. The TC attempted to dictate a new perspective on resident's past lives, one which viewed them as wholly negative and without any redeeming worth. In the TC code, residents were labeled "dope fiends," characterized as frequently ill or otherwise incapacitated. The high of heroin was defined as an unfeeling stupor, a flight from authentic human feelings. While many residents accepted the characterization of their prior lives as destructive, residents generally remembered the herion experience itself as pleasurable. Eight of the 19 residents offered unsolicited testimonies to the inherent appeal of heroin long after detoxification. Only one ex-heroin user claimed to be "burned out" on the drug. These findings confirm that of Carlson (1976: 579). In this TC, a resident highly placed in the status structure, and about to enter the re-entry portion of the program, spoke of the good times he had throughout a period of extremely heavy drug abuse and heroin addiction. When asked by the observer what he wanted to do upon graduation, his response was that he wanted to "party." He said he did not want to give up the life of good times associated with drug use. Residents also discussed the rewards of street life, including money and prestige, (see e.g., Lindesmith (1968), Preble and Casey (1969), and Stephens and McBride (1976).)

How are these violations of TC rules to be understood? Becker (1960) has advanced the concept of side bets to explain actions which appear unexpectedly in the context. He views these actions as consistent with another perspective in which the actor maintains some investment. TC residents' "war stories" can be viewed as side bets in the values of the drug subculture maintained in spite of the immediate risks associated with such behavior in the TC. Perhaps by telling "war stories," residents reassured themselves that the most meaningful act of their prior lives, the procurement and use of drugs, was not the unmitigated squalor depicted in the TC interpretation. This reassurance may have been an important bit of personal insurance for residents who were aware that they might easily return to their past lives where they would again have to apply the skills of the street hustler.

Even those residents who expressed personal commitments to new lives were aware of the odds against total rehabilitation. Many had stayed clean on their own for sustained periods only to return to addiction. Evaluation studies have confirmed that long-term residential treatment is consistently related to reductions in rates of drug use, criminal arrests, convictions, and incarceration, as well as to increased employment following treatment (Aron & Daily, 1974; Bale et al., 1980; Barr et al., 1973; Biase, 1972; De Leon et al., 1979; De Leon, et al., 1982; Chambers & Inciardi, 1974; Coombs, 1981; Simpson, et al., 1979; Wilson & Mandelbrote, 1978). Nevertheless, clients were not sanguine about their own futures. Within the TC, split rates (voluntary departure prior to graduation) were high, and, in the TC folklore shared by residents, graduates who re-entered the community and stayed clean were thought to be rare. Residents were familiar with stories of ex-addict TC staff members who had returned to drugs after long periods as drug abstinent counselors. Residents had no guarantees that they would remain drug free when they returned to the outside would. A senior resident talked to the observer of having solved many personal problems while in the TC, but of having no assurance that he would be able to stay away from alcohol and heroin after leaving.

It is interesting to note that one of the most sustained sharings of "war stories" was observed among senior members of the treatment status struture. While on a vacation retreat conducted by the TC, five residents discussed the pros and cons of street life. They debated the comparative material rewards of straight and street life. They weighed probabilities of arrest and spoke of the "rush" of hustling. This group was on a verge of entry into the re-entry component of the program. A return to street life and drug use was one of the possible futures for such residents. By telling "war stories" of their prowess on the streets and tales of their drug exploits, residents could reassure themselves that the drug life had its own rewards and that they had the skills to return to it and survive if they relapsed after leaving the TC. By telling "war stories," they made side bets on their street skills even as they participated in TC treatment.

One resident's case is illustrative. At one point he described his life on the street:

> I wasn't functioning anymore, I was back in prison after a month out here and a month out there, and I was doing crazier and crazier things to buy drugs. I started to realize I couldn't shoot drugs or I'd be in prison for the rest of my life. But if anyone tells me there is any feeling in the world better than shooting heroin, they're either ignorant or they're lying.

Subsequently, this resident told the observer while in the community on an errand, that the only thing preventing him from leaving and procuring a bag of heroin at that moment was the presence of the observer. He boasted that he would "cop a big in 20 minutes and someone between here and there would be out of the money." The resident made these remarks moments after someone he identified as a former "running partner" had driven by the corner on which the resident and observer was standing. This resident used a moment of sanctuary outside the TC to exercise an image of himself as a strong-arm hustler, perhaps as a side bet on his ability to survive on the streets again if necessary, in spite of his verbal commitment to changing his life through TC treatment. Perhaps equally important was the payoff in self-esteem from this opportunity to make a positive self-assertion and describe a coherent personal history with points of reference that exceeded the temporally limited perspectives of the TC.

Using Institutional Mechanisms to Make Secondary Adjustments

We have suggested some possible reasons that TC residents talk of their drug experiences and street exploits in spite of the inherent risks associated with such behavior in the TC. Often there is a double movement of simultaneous compliance with TC expectations and participation in telling the forbidden war stories. Given the encompassing character of the mechanisms TCs use to control behavior, how do residents get away with such behavior? Interestingly, in this TC, often the very mechanisms of the pullup system facilitated such secondary adjustments.

As incessant peer monitoring became part of everyday life, residents developed an acute awareness of the behavior of other residents and staff, and their physical dispositions in the TC. This awareness was coupled with a hightened sensitivity to the boundaries of personal space and the limits of surveillance. This heightened space-time awareness, in fact, provided residents with a tool for making secondary adjustments. Residents became so attuned to patterns of surveillance that they identified lapses in surveillance as free spaces in which they could carry on interpersonal business not sanctioned by the TC. In effect, they created sanctuaries in the midst of their fellow residents.

This phenomenon was first voluntered to the observer by a resident who suggested he note how residents related to each other on free time when they were "being real." She said that residents created considerable physical space for themselves by using living room couches in a certain way. She described, and the observer later confirmed, instances in which residents sat close to each other in the center of the couch, thereby creating considerable "dead space" which would deter other clients from approaching the conversation and preclude eavesdropping. According to the informant, once having set up in this way, residents carried on conversations about forbidden topics. Conversation began only when considerable space was cleared by the preoccupation and inattention of other residents.

A systematic body language was used in over 60 "setups" of this kind witnessed by the observer. Residents leaned backward, their legs extended before them, and extended one arm along the back or seat of the couch. This configuration produced an apparent openness which paradoxically precluded any approach but the most visible to the heart of the space. Some speakers guarded against interpretation of facial gestures by adopting a deadpan expression. One resident used the fall of long hair and the habital placement of a hand over her mouth to screen out observers. Others tilted their heads in ways which also subtly obscured significant facial expressions.

Maintaining a setup required subtle awareness of how the conversation would appear to fellow residents. Any conspicuous intimacy might be confronted by other clients as a "negative hookup" or a "contract" (a personal compact between residents to circumvent the TC code), so minute changes in the disposition of other residents sometimes ended conversations which might appear to have gone on too long. The observer attempted on 15 occasions to approach one of these conversations without interrupting. The observer met with no success even when approaching clients with whom he had established rapport. The observer also witnessed over 20 instances in the four-week period when the approach of a client into such spaces ended conversations. The observer participated in two such conversations with one client where an extended metaphor (that of a chess game) adopted by the client was used to shield a discussion of TC interpersonal dynamics from eavesdroppers. Ultimately, the observer was able to use these sanctuaries to talk with residents anxious about confiding sensitive information. In two cases, when a resident became anxious about continuing the conversation, the observer urged the resident to check whether anyone else in the room was tuned in. In both instances, the resident did so by relaxing a moment as if taking a deep breath, taking a measured look about the room, then calmly returned to the topic of discussion.

Residents used a number of other mechanisms to create "free spaces" for themselves. For example, as they carried out daily chores, residents were expected to constantly discuss the TC ideology (called "kicking the concept"). In this way, the TC demanded a constant obligatory engrossment of both mind and body (Goffman, 1961:176). Failure to "kick the concept" was to be met with a pullup. While on work details, residents used the background noise of portable radios either to mask their conversations regarding illicit topics or to evade their responsibility for "kicking the concept." This "free space" was equally important in creating individual privacy for residents to engage in moments of introspection, forbidden, and to a large extent structured out, by the TC schedule of seminars, rap sessions, group therapy, and constant surveillance.

Residents also learned to use closed areas, such as laundry rooms and maintenance sheds, set apart from the major centers of activity, as sanctuaries for conversations free from the oversight of others. One resident spoke of the maintenance shed as a place where people could "kick back and have a smoke break" without being overseen. On three occasions, the observer was party to underlife conversations in this area. Topics of conversation included prison experiences, street hustling, and shared fantasies of drug use after leaving the TC. Residents also used this sanctuary to complain about the boredom of work assignments and to indulge in mild forms of criticism of the program and other residents outside of group sessions. A resident also reported to the observer a conversation about procuring heroin that took place between the informant and another resident in this area.

Limiting the Impact of Institutional Mechanisms

At first glance, institutional mechanisms such as pullups appear encompassing and overwhelming. We have seen, however, that they also serve to heighten residents' awareness of opportunities for carrying out forbidden activities. Further, we have seen how residents in this TC used these opportunities to engage in secondary adjustments. Residents were also able to minimize that impact of institutional mechanisms by selecting the instances in which these mechanisms were employed.

Goffman has pointed out that total institutions demand "obligatory engrossment" of residents. "Part of the individual's obligation is to be visibly engaged in the activity of the organization" (1961:176). Giving a pullup in a TC acts as a symbol of commitment to the program, an advertisment that the resident is participating in the therapy of fellow residents. Yet, by limiting use of the pullups to certain situations and types of behavior, residents were able to advertise involvement while minimizing the likelihood that pullups had the effect intended.

In the TC discussed here, this was accomplished by limiting the use of pullups to the most physically obvious lapses of time-space awareness and not using them in instances of more serious, but less immediately obvious, violations of program rules.

During the month's residence in the TC, the observer recorded up to 40 pullups a day given for lapses of time-space awareness including leaving tools and personal property out of place, leaving cups unattended, dropping silverware, and less than perfectly made beds. Each of these violations was easily observed and identified. Residents who observed such an event and failed to give a pullup for it put themselves at risk, for such events were often observed by others who easily recognized them as appropriate for pullups. Failure to use the pullup in such situations could result in a confrontation during group.

On the other hand, the observer documented 18 incidents in which residents violated rules regarding interpersonal interactions, yet received no pullups from other residents for these violations. In addition, on 13 different occasions, evidence emerged in group sessions that residents had failed to use pullups in similar situations. These instances in which pullups were not given included cases in which residents discussed their feelings about other residents outside the group, told "war stories" or spoke on other forbidden topics, or evidenced negative attitudes toward the TC or their work responsibilities.

This selective use of pullups minimized their impact on both those who would give and those eligible to receive them. While being confronted for a lapse of time and space awareness may threaten a person's self-image, confrontation for such a behavior is likely to be less threatening than to be confronted for an emotional state, the content of one's conversation, or one's attitude. Thus, choosing to confront for a lapse in space-time awareness was choosing a focus of attack which was less personally threatening to the one confronted. This choice also minimized risk to the potential pullup giver. Pullups could be discussed and challenged in group sessions. People who gave pullup based on the judgment that someone had a negative attitude could be called on in group to defend the charge, to point to the evidence, and even to show that they had not simply expressed their own negative feelings about the person confronted through use of the pullup. Giving a pullup for an emotional state or for content of a conversation risked much more than to give a pullup for a lapse in space-time awareness.

Residents of this TC learned how to work a tight and encompassing system. They learned to use pullups selectively, thereby manifesting the "obligatory engrossment" demanded by the TC self-help ideology while at the same time using the heightened awareness generated by the pullup system to secure time and space to engage in conversations about forbidden topics. In so doing, they were able to minimize the risks of TC sanctions which could accompany these secondary adjustments.

Discussion

TCs, like other total institutions, are encompassing. They direct the lives of residents while in residence. Conventional friendships, sexual contact, introspection, and association with the outside world are all forbidden. Yet most TCs are not total in one important dimension: the temporal one. With several notable exceptions, such as Synanon and monasteries, these institutions ultimately intend to return their residents to the outside world. Residents know they will return to this world some day. Even while inside, they look to this return. More importantly, they prepare for it (Wheeler, 1961).

Secondary adjustments among residents of total institutions may indicate their efforts to prepare for return to the outside society. In the TC case we have examined, residents' preparations for return to the larger society appear to include telling "war stories" of their prowess on the streets and sharing accounts of the pleasures and rewards of the drug experience and lifestyle. Residents are aware that the changes made in the TC may last after they leave. They have evidence from prior residents which confirms these doubts. In this situation, there preparations for life after the TC may include risking the immediate sanctions of TC to make a side bet on both the rewards of the street life and their skills to obtain these rewards. Some residents appear to make such side bets even as they work toward the rehabilitation offered by the TC.

A recognition of the temporary hold total institutions have on their residents increases the plausibility of the suggestion that secondary adjustments such as "war stories" in TCs may be side bets made on residents' abilities to make it when they return to the outside world. This suggestion does not imply that the high incidence of conventional and prosocial behavior in TCs is simple compliance or the equivalent of "doing time." Simultaneous participation in the world of the TC and the world of "war stories" may be adaptive behavior, with the side bet on street life serving as a kind of disaster insurance against the possibility of relapse even as residents strive to master the skills of conventional life.

If our interpretations are correct, their implications for TC therapy are important. TCs appear generally successful in helping residents develop new self-identities which do not depend on the addict habits of exploitation, dishonesty, or insensitivity to others. Some TCs have implemented treatment as if this resocialization is the major change necessary to ensure success in the larger society. Perhaps resocialization is only one step, however important, in the process of rehabilitation of drug abusers.

TCs may have to undertake two major additional tasks. The first is to deal directly and honestly with residents' fears of failure in the community rather than trying to suppress conversations about street exploits. It is probably both wasteful and dysfunctional to try to totally eliminate side bets residents make on their abilities to survive after treatment. Rather, discussions with residents should recognize the attraction of the street life itself. Drug abusers are not merely crazed, immature "dope fiends." Their prior lives were not exclusively squalor and sickness. Street life offered excitement, money, prestige, and independence as well as problems. To openly discuss these realities and residents' desires to return to the excitement while fearing the addiction and hassle which led them to the TC in the first place clearly is a challenge to TC staffs. Yet dealing openly and directly with residents' fears of failure and their desires for the benefits of the drug life may enable residents to develop realistic expectations for their posttreatment lives. It may also aid in identifying the skills necessary to survive on the outside without a return to drugs.

The rehabilitated individual who leaves TC treatment is not a superhuman creature who can make it alone on the strength of character generated in a TC. Former TC residents need a number of additional practical skills. The second major task facing TCs may be to engage in extensive skills training for residents. These should include the skills necessary to find and hold work worth more to the former resident than the exciting and often lucrative scale of drugs. Residents will also need to learn the skills to recognize moments of crisis in daily life which they will inevitably face and the skills to secure appropriate assistance in weathering these. Further, they will need to learn the skills to **control** drug use should they slip into it, rather than labeling themselves as failures doomed to readdiction if they slip. Finally, residents will need to learn skills to develop and maintain informal social support systems whose members share the values and perspectives created in the TC. Teaching residents these additional skills will not be easy. Yet, when TCs do not provide these practical skills needed to survive without drugs following treatment, TC residents are likely to make side bets on their survival skills as street hustlers both during and after treatment.

CHAPTER 13

MOTIVATIONAL ASPECTS OF HEROIN ADDICTS IN THERAPEUTIC COMMUNITIES COMPARED WITH THOSE IN OTHER INSTITUTIONS

DAGMAR ZIMMER-HOFLER

PETER MEYER-FEHR

1. Introduction

THE SCIENTIFIC literature about the outcome of heroin addicts has increased considerably during the last years. Some classical studies were pioneers (Vaillant, 1962 and 1973; Wimick, 1962; Glasscote, 1972; De Leon et al., 1972; and others). In the meantime, a quite sophisticated literature has developed telling young researchers how to do those studies and what methods and techniques are advisable (Maddoux and Desmond, 1975; Bale and Cabrera, 1977; Platt et al., 1977; Kandel, 1978). Small and large national programs in the United States (Sells et al., 1976) and Europe (SNF, 1977) have been established to investigate the issues of addiction and treatment outcome. Even small institutions and workers in the field are encouraged to evaluate their work (Johnston et al., 1977).

While it is favorable to see this increase in research in order to deliver facts and knowledge for the general and political discussion about addiction and its treatment, there are dangers in it as well. The worst danger being that research remains meaningless for practical use.

The task for researchers is to find the right form of communication. During fieldwork, they have to stay in contact with the addicts and the staff (Zimmer-Hofler, 1981) and afterwards, to be able to communicate their results in an understandable way (Zimmer-Hofler & Meyer-Fehr, 1983).

157

The task for the TC is to accept the findings of research and be ready to alter prejudices and attitudes and to renounce an ideological over-identified and narrow-minded approach to their work. This is not at all easy. We have pointed out elsewhere (Zimmer-Hofler & Widmer, 1981b) the tendency of therapeutic communities to overestimate their own concept or program and devaluate those of others. This is also a problem with other programs working with addicted persons. Addiction itself seems to have an intrinsic effect of polarization which is called by Petzold (1980) pathological confluence and is understandable in its psychodynamics.

This is still an immature feature which can change during the rehabilitation. We think it is important to control these impulses in ourselves and not to act them out if we are staff, administrators or researchers in an institution working with addicts. Research can be a very good tool to help us in this respect. The question is: Can the researcher provide the tools and if so, will the staff want to use them?

2. Research Questions

Research questions prestructure to some extent what will be seen. There we have to be distrustful and precautious, just like non-researchers are towards use. Especially in the field of psychosocial science, we should first know for whom our work is intended and in which soil the seeds of our findings will fall. We should be personally touched and develop our intuition to ask the right questions.

The research questions we want to follow in this article are not focussing on outcome; this will be done later elsewhere. We want to look at some aspects of motivation concerning the resident's **readiness to renounce drugs** (DVB) and his **orientation for the future** (ZOR). We will look at different programs or institutions with regard to these points and also consider interfering variables, e.g., voluntariness of entry and participation in the program.

Then we will look at their relationship with the "time-in-program" (De Leon, 1973, 1979), called by us in the tables BEHDAU, according to the German expression "Behandlungsdauer."

Another aspect is the motivation for the program which we call "**compliance**." Finally we want to look at the **social climate** in different therapeutic communities, in terms of our conceptualization, described earlier with empiric methods.

We can formulate our questions as follows:

2.1 Do the aspects of motivation which we call readiness to renounce drugs (DVB) and orientation for the future (ZOR), differ across various therapeutic communitites compared to methadone- programs or addicts in prison?

2.2 Does time-in-program influence these aspects of motivation and does it relate to the voluntariness of treatment-participation?

2.3 Which interactions exist between the described variables and the voluntariness of entry and participation in the program?

2.4. How does the motivation and compliance for the program differ in different residential institutions, e.g., different therapeutic communities and how far does compliance depend on the climate?

3. Methods

The data we present here are from a research project of the Social Psychiatric Service of the Psychiatric University Hospital of Zurich (Uchtenhagen and Zimmer-Hofler, 1983), which is part of the mentioned National Research Program "Social Integration" of the Swiss National Research Fund. The study included a very thorough face-to-face interview with heroin addicts in different institutions, a follow-up interview after 2-3 years, an analysis of the therapeutic institutions and a comparative study with a matched representative normal control group derived from a representative study of the same program with comparable items (Blacpain et al., 1983). The special aspects of interviewing heroin addicts for research are presented elsewhere (Zimmer-Hofler, 1981).

The data we present in the following are from the first interview with addicts in different institutions and from the analysis of the therapeutic institutions. The statistical procedures to analyze the data will be mentioned with the presentation of the results; they are all part of the SPSS-System (Statistical Package for Social Science) and were carried out at the center for electronic data-analysis (Rechenzentrum) of the University of Zurich, Switzerland.

4. Results

4.1 Readiness to Renounce Drugs (DVB) and Orientation for the Future (ZOR) in Different Institutions

Out of different items, measuring these variables, an index was constructed which could be scaled from 1 to 10. The highest score would be

10, the lowest 1. Results were obtained on the mean-values of the analysis of variance for consensual therapeutic communities (including democratic, family-type and religious concepts), hierarchical therapeutic communities, methadone programs and prison.

The two measured aspects of motivation are quite high in all programs. Highest is the readiness to renounce drugs in the consensual TCs; 2nd is the orientation for the future in the methadone programs and 3rd is the orientation for the future in the consensual TCs, almost equally scaling with the readiness to renounce drugs of the methadone patients. In the 5th place ranges the readiness to renounce drugs in the hierarchical TC and 6th the orientation for the future there. The orientation for the future of imprisoned addicts takes the 7th place and their readiness to renounce drugs takes place 8. It is interesting that in both drugfree residential groups, the readiness to renounce drugs (DVB) ranges higher than the orientation for the future (ZOR), but in methadone and prison it is reversed. This seems to express a different motivational pattern, though we do not know whether it implies a different population or the adaption to the aims of the programs.

Results also show that the two measured variables are in a significantly close relationship with each other in all groups, but somewhat less in prison.

From Table 1 we see that the distribution of the mean values (of analysis of variance) over the compared groups differs significantly, more so for the readiness to renounce drugs (DVB) and, still significant, but less for the orientation for the future (ZOR). We also see how the compared institutions differ for the **voluntariness of entering** the program. It can hardly be expected that addicts entered prison voluntarily and our investigation reveals that only 5 percent entered the hierarchical TC by free decision.

In the consensual TCs almost 70 percent are there on their free decision. The methadone program has the highest rate with almost 84 percent. The voluntariness of participation reveals that therapeutic communities, including the hierarchically structured, have a strong motivating aspect compared to methadone and prison. But still the prison has succeeded to motivate about 20 percent of the residents for voluntary participation. The last column shows final court decision which is the highest in the hierarchical TC, lower in prison, because half of those residents were still in detention there. In the methadone program the punishment seems to be given in most cases after the program was voluntarily entered.

Table 1

DIFFERENCES OF THE VARIABLES "READINESS TO RENOUNCE ON DRUGS" (DVB), "ORIENTATION FOR THE FUTURE" (ZOR), "VOLUNTARITY OF ENTERING THE PROGRAM" (FREIE2), "VOLUNTARITY OF PARTICIPATION (FREIT2) AND "SELF-REPORTED FINAL COURT DECISIONS" (DETOSA2).

Typology of institutions ST4A	N	Analysis of variance mean-values of categories		From crosstabs		
		DVB	ZOR	FREIE2 %	FREIT2 %	DETOSA2 %
hierarchical TC	58	6.65	6.14	5%	67%	86%
consensual TC	32	8.67	6.90	69%	100%	41%
prison (detention) (executive inprisonment)	53	5.83	5.96	0%	19%	66%
methadone (outpatients)	63	6.89	7.01	84%	76%	43%
Total	206	6.83	6.48	38%	63%	61%
Analysis of variance:						
Eta		.42	.24			
F, significance		14.5 ***	4.3 **			
Crosstabs:						
Cramer's V, significance				.79***	.57***	.38***

Mark to the level of significance: ***: 0.1%, **: 1%, *: 5%

These data indicate that the residents of the hierarchical TC are at their start-off-point in terms of voluntary motivation the closest to the imprisoned addicts. If we compare both, then the motivational structure is different and both values are higher. The question arises, whether this is a result of the treatment or a pre-existing feature in terms of spontaneous selection of the residents.

We approach the answer by observing that there is highly significant correlation of the DVB with BEHDAU in the therapeutic communities (+ 0.47), while no such correlation is obtained in the methadone program and a slightly negative correlation in the prison. This means that only therapeutic communities have a socializing influence on the motivation of addicts to renounce drugs. This influence correlates with the time-in-program. We have also checked the influence of voluntary entrance of the program and found that the longer the time-in-program endures, the less relevant the original voluntariness becomes and finally loses all relevance.

We can conclude that addicts in therapeutic communities of either type show a strongly positive development in readiness to renounce drugs and orientation for the future, independent of the voluntariness of entering the program, but highly dependent on the time-in-program.

Patients in the methadone program seem to enter the program with a quite high motivation in both of the investigated aspects, but do not improve. The program may help them realize their orientation for the future which is the leading motivational aspect.

The worst situation is shown by the imprisoned addicts. They have the least motivation in both aspects and tend to be reduced the longer they stay. Since the time-in-program proved again to be relevant variable, more detailed results and tables are contained in a German article (Meyer-Fehr and Zimmer-Hofler, 1983a).

4.2 Compliance and Motivation for Different Institutions

The results of another evaluation of our data (Meyer-Fehr and Zimmer-Hofler, 1983b) reveal a similar difference between the therapeutic community and the prison. We excluded methadone programs because of their different institutional conditions.

We wanted to investigate the motivation for the program and called this aspect "compliance" according to Etzioni (1961 and 1964). Etzioni differentiates three types of compliance:

☐ the moral orientation and positive identification with the institution
☐ the calculating orientation with a relatively indifferent attitude towards the institution
☐ the alineated orientation with refusing or rejecting attitude.

For our evaluations, we summarize the three types into two: The identification (with the residence, the program, the peergroup, the staff) which we call **positive compliance,** and the criticism and rejection which we call **negative compliance.**

We obtained significant differences for the positive identification with their stay-in-the-program and the type of program itself. This is not as astonishing as the fact that only 30 percent of the residents in prison identify themselves with their stay and about 25 percent with the institution. The peergroup has the most important identification in TCs and in prison and shows no differences. It is the most important aspect of positive compliance in prison. The identification with the staff is low in TCs and in prison, shows no statistical difference, but is a bit higher in prison. There the question arises, whether this indicates a special sub-group of addicts relating to staff or parental figures, which we cannot answer here. Criticism of the program is higher in prison, but does not show statistical program differences and rejection does differ significantly.

Comparisons across different concepts of therapeutic communities gives an interesting result. We see a kind of spectrum, ranging from the highest positive compliance and the lowest negative compliance in the religious TC in steps to the lowest positive, and the highest negative compliance in detention (religious TC = 1st place, detention, TC last = 5th place). The second place in this spectrum is taken by the democratic TC, the third by the hierarchical TC and the fourth by executive imprisonment.

In all institutions there is a high identification with the peergroup (slightly lower in the democratic TC). This further proves the importance of peers in the rehabilitation of addicts, but we are worried about the influence the peergroup may have in prison. This might explain the negative correlation of the readiness to renounce drugs with the duration of imprisonment.

We see that in the hierarchical TC there is the highest peergroup identification and the lowest staff identification that corresponds with the conceptual goals. It also shows how much responsibility is given to the senior residents and that their role modeling has to be well controlled.

An unexpected result is the relatively higher identification with the resident in executive imprisonment corresponding with a relatively lower rejection. We could ask, whether this means that these addicts show a sense of justice, or that they are glad not to be in a TC, or that they just feel safe and protected there.

Summarizing the results from this evaluation, we can say that, in comparison to prisons, therapeutic communities show a remarkable ability to motivate residents positively for their program.

Within the varieties of therapeutic communities a range can be observed with the highest positive and the lowest negative compliance in the religious community and with the relatively lowest positive and relatively highest negative compliance in the hierarchical TC. The democratic concept is in between. This goes along with the time-in-program, the voluntariness of residence and the size of the institutions, but in this evaluation we did not investigate the possible interactions (Zimmer-Hofler et al., 1982).

The data this far analyzed are from the first resident interview of our follow-up and career study, and they show different motivational aspects of therapeutic communities (TCs) in comparison to methadone programs and prisons. Compared with those institutions, TCs appear rather homogeneous, but if we focus on the differences between various concepts of TC's, we see that they are different not only in aspects of motivation, but also involuntariness. Thus it seems to be of some interest to look at the data stemming from the analysis of therapeutic communities, including staff and residents, which was collected two years later in the same institutions (enlarged by a few more of each type). From these additional empirical aspects, we want to contribute to the description of the different TC-concepts.

Since the social surrounding is a main issue for the rehabilitation of addicts in therapeutic communities, an analysis of the social atmosphere can be usefully investigated.

The Social Atmosphere Scale was originally introduced by Moos (1974) and the modified one by a German group (Henrich, 1979). We used the version of Henrich et al. and adapted it for our needs. More details are given in scientific report (Meyer-Fehr and Zimmer-Hofler, 1983b).

We think the scale is also quite useful as a feedback to the institution and could be part of dynamic self-evaluation and self-control of the social climate. We have pointed out these possibilities before (Zimmer-Hofler and Meyer-Fehr, 1983b) and want to repeat only the most interesting results here and then show some further steps that we have taken in the analysis of these data.

The judgement of the social climate were obtained from residents and staff in different concepts of TCs. All four types of TCs differ significantly in the judgement of their own concept. The 15 scales consisting each of 5 or 4 items can be summarized to four dimensions which are the "participation of the residents," the "conception of the program," the "functioning of the program" and the "inter-staff-relationship."

The differences are all highly significant and prove again the spectrum we have seen already concerning the compliance. It is important to mention that these data are taken from the same (and a few more) communities about two years after the compliance research.

In most items the religious TC scores the highest values. The lowest ones are scored by the hierarchical TC in most items. On the second place values for most items are scored by the family-type concept and somewhat more inconsistently the third place is taken by the democratic TC which scores higher than the religious for "resident's spontaneity," lower than the hierarchical for "preparation for the future" (of the program) and lowest of all for "staff control."

Additionally, we found that staff and residents perceive differently the social atmosphere; staff tend to overestimate the quality of the social atmosphere, residents score mostly lower. This is very significant in hierarchical TCs, less in the consensual TCs where in some items residents even score a little bit higher. The biggest gap occurs in the conceptualization of the program, where in hierarchical TCs, especially the "therapeutic modeling," the "preparation for the future" (which the concept delivers), and the "reinforcement" are overestimated by the staff (or underestimated by the residents). But we think the resident's perception should be taken seriously, because, if they do not get the message, they can not adapt it.

We tried to reduce the information through factor analysis of the scales and correlating these with type of TC. The factor analysis (further description: see Meyer-Fehr and Zimmer-Hofler 1983) revealed three factors, explaining 62 percent of the total variance of the 15 scales.

Factor 1, "relationship": describes a spontaneous egalitarian quality of the relationship.

Factor 2, "therapy": describes a therapeutic conception which is based on practical considerations and necessities for the future and fosters the autonomy of the residents.

Factor 3, "order": describes a well organized program led by staff who serve as a role model.

The results of the factor analysis showed that staff and residents in all TC-concepts judge the quality of the relationships identically.

The **relationships** in the democratic TCs are judged to be of the highest quality. Those in family-type or religious TCs range much lower and in the hierarchical relationships are TCs lowest.

This seems to be a contradiction to our aforementioned spectrum, but it is explained by the fact that the scale control correlates high, but negatively with this factor and is part of it. Thus a lower value results for the religious- and family-type concepts with a significant correlation, in spite of the high values for relationship in the earlier analyses on social climate.

The lowest range is taken as before by the hierarchical TC. The factor **therapy** reveals that staff judges the realization of their therapeutic concepts to be much better than the residents do. Hierarchical and democratic TCs have the worst conceptualization in terms of this factor. The family-type TC scores rather high and the religious TC the highest.

The factor **order** is mostly considered by the staff to be higher than it is by the clients. The highest scores for this factor are to be found in the religious TC. In the hierarchical and family-type, this factor scores closely to the mean values, but the democratic concept scores much lower. They have the worst order and organization and the staff does not serve in their opinion as role model in this respect which might be part of the ideology.

5. What Do We Derive from These Studies?

We proposed a research approach which would produce understandable information for everybody interested in the subject. At the same time we want to encourage discussion and consider research not as a dogma, but as a contribution. In this sense we shall try to conclude some main results.

5.1 The readiness to renounce drugs and the orientation for the future are closely related. The relationship is most pronounced in therapeutic communities, second in methadone programs, least in prison.

5.2 In therapeutic communities the readiness to renounce drugs is highly dependent on time-in-program. The longer residents spent in TCs the less important the fact of voluntary or involuntary entrance in the program becomes. The time-in-program correlates also with a higher readiness to renounce drugs than with the voluntariness to participate in the program.

5.3 In methadone programs the readiness to renounce drugs does not have any correlation with time spent in a program. Methadone seems to have well motivated clients with respect to their social reintegration. This seems to be like this from the beginning and does not change during the program. Thus the contribution of the methadone program might be to give the clients a chance to realize their intentions to reintegrate themselves.

5.4 With imprisoned addicts the readiness to renounce drugs does not change considerably, it can even be reduced during their stay in prison.

5.5 The socializing influence of therapeutic communities is even more remarkable since it is also true for involuntary residents. This suggests that it is better to send addicts to TCs rather than to prison for executive punishment.

5.6 The motivation for the institution, which we call compliance, shows similiar connections like those described for the personal motivation of the addicts. We can observe a spectrum with the most positive and the least negative compliance in the TCs according to the following order: 1. religious TCs; 2. family-type TCs; 3. democratic; and 4. hierarchic TCs. The prisons have, however, high values for the negative and low for the positive compliance. Even though it is remarkable and unexpected, there is also positive compliance found by some addicts.

5.7 The analysis of the therapeutic climate shows a verification of the "spectrum" by new data in a more detailed investigation. Ranging in the first place, with the best climate (according to the self-judgment of clients and staff), is again the religious TC; in the second place the family-type TC (which we did not investigate in the compliance-study), in third place the democratic, and in fourth place the hierarchical TCs.

5.8 Staff and residents judge the aspects of the therapeutic conception quite differently and as a rule the staff overestimates it in comparison with the residents, especially in hierarchical TCs.

5.9 Factor-analysis gives a new perspective of the social climate. Three factors can be identified: "relationship," "therapy" and "order." Democratic TCs judge the factor "relationship" to be of the highest quality (in terms of intimacy). The lowest judgement for this factor is seen in hierarchical TCs. Religious and family-type TCs are in between. For "therapy" and "order," however, religious and family-type TCs score highest (religious even a bit higher), hierarchic and democratic both low in comparison, but democratic lowest.

All results indicate that therapeutic communities, of any conception are, for the motivating and socializing aspects, superior to imprisonment and also to the methadone program.

We can see also that those TCs which are primarily non-therapeutic, but defined as social structures range higher. They show better compliance and also higher values for the factors "therapy" and "order." It is difficult to distinguish how much the family-structure and how much the religious background contribute to this fact, because the religious TCs we investigated were also based on a family-structure.

Democratic and hierarchical concepts are both lower for the two mentioned factors and relatively close together. However, they differ considerably for the factor "relationship." Here the democratic one ranges highest and hierarchical lowest. This could be the explanation for the described polarization. The intimacy of relationship between therapists and patients is a main issue for all therapeutic schools and a very provoking and controversal topic of discussion. It could also relate to what we have pointed out before as "pathological confluence" (Petzold, 1980) either acting it out in close intimacy or forming a reaction with too rigid structures and control.

But the natural development can get lost in their solution which is then of no practical use for the residents. In the first place they need, in order to develop, reliable, mature role models and supporting social structures which are as natural as possible. Probably, that is primarily what all therapeutic concepts can learn from the religious or the family-type TC: It is practicing structure, order and ideals of life and not mere preaching them that finally counts.

CHAPTER 14

MEASURING PROCESS IN DRUG ABUSE TREATMENT RESEARCH

SHERRY HOLLAND*

INTRODUCTION

THIS CHAPTER presents a framework for describing treatments in drug abuse research, with special reference to residential drug free programs (Therapeutic Communities). At present, studies of drug abuse interventions provide little or no information about the treatments being studied. Readers of a study on program X, for example, may learn only that program X is a "classical therapeutic community." Such "standard treatment" labels mask wide variations among programs in actual organization, clientele, and procedures. Reporting treatment effectiveness without specifying the treatment provided has been compared to reporting on the efficacy of a drug without specifying the quantity, frequency and total time the drug has been administered. Even when the "same" drug is prescribed to different people, the prescribed strength may vary (Sechrest and Redner, 1979).

The primary reason to measure treatments is that variations in the nature and level of program activity may be associated with differences in outcomes. By studying the relationships among variations in treatment parameters and outcome, we can identify more precisely what it is about treatments that allow people to change. In addition, detailed information about treatments is necessary to facilitate comparisons of outcomes across studies, to permit the pooling of findings from studies of similar treatments, and to estimate the replicability of treatments.

*This research was supported in part by a grant from the Dr. Scholl Foundation.

Describing drug abuse interventions is not easy. Such treatments often are very complex, with multiple change-induction techniques being used to impact multiple target behaviors. Also, with the notable exception of the work of Moos and his colleagues, very little spadework has been done in this area. There is no "how to" book on measuring treatment. Attention in the past 15 years has focused on identifying and measuring client variables. While the work on client attributes is critical, similar effort needs to be applied to problem of explicating the treatment construct.

The descriptive framework presented in this chapter is based on the premise that there are multiple users of treatment information, and that potential users may need data at the micro (procedures) or macro (clinics or system) level. The objective of the framework is to produce a profile of a treatment clinic or unit which can be summarized with other clinic profiles to describe a system or disaggregated into information about procedures. The profile consists of three classes of questions most frequently asked about treatment: 1) organizational structure, such as location, size, and costs; 2) the nature of the client population; and 3) the nature of the treatment process, or what is done to bring about intended changes. These classes of questions will be briefly discussed below, although emphasis will be placed upon treatment process in residential settings.

By treatment "process" we mean the activities, procedures, and techniques which programs undertake to produce specified changes in target individuals. These process variables, or "inputs," may be conceptualized in terms of discrete "services," such as group counseling, as well as in terms of interactions among clients and staff which take place during and outside of such scheduled activities. Inputs may also include less interpersonal procedures such as prescribing medication as part of the treatment plan.

By means of organizational parameters — e.g., physical setting, primary orientation, use of medication — programs can be grouped into a relatively small number of program "types." For example, organizational variables have been used to create a typology consisting of four "major modalities": detoxification, maintenance, outpatient drug-free, and residential drug-free. Such a typology makes possible certain preliminary analyses relating outcomes to gross program differences. In addition, however, the operations of programs within each type will vary greatly. This systematic variation in the nature and intensity of program activity allows for comparative research on the "active ingredients" in treatment. If the things that programs do cause people to change, variations in the patterns and strength of these activities should be associated with differential impact on target behaviors.

Target behaviors, or treatment "outputs," are the attitudes, cognitions, feelings and behaviors which treatment programs attempt to add to, change, or eliminate from clients' repertoires. Treatment outputs can be divided into intermediate objectives and end goals. End goals are those criterion outcomes which drug rehabilitation programs typically are mandated to effect, such as reduction or elimination of drug use and criminality, and an increase in productive employment. Of course, programs may posit other goals for their clients. Intermediate objectives are those changes which programs believe are necessary to achieve in order to attain and maintain end goals.

Implicit in what programs do are causal theories relating inputs and outputs. These theories can be simple or complex. For example, an early hypothesis regarding the relationship between methadone maintenance and criminality stated that, since drug abusers commit crimes in order to buy drugs, providing abusers with free drugs will eliminate criminal behaviors. A more complex theory assumes that criminal behavior is multi-determined. Drug abusers commit crimes not only to buy drugs but also to buy food, clothes, and to pay the rent; because it is acceptable, even "normal" behavior; because it is the only thing they know how to do; because it is exciting. According to this theory, in order to eliminate criminal behavior it is necessary to change several mediating variables, e.g., change attitudes, teach job skills, teach people how to enjoy themselves in "pro-social" ways.

One can describe process variables without describing target behaviors and the program's assumptions about how treatment inputs and outputs are related. However, for reasons which may already be obvious, a process description which also specifies what outcomes are anticipated, and why, is significantly more useful than one which focuses only on planned inputs. By explicating the theory, we specify key questions to address as well as the relevant program content to measure. If a program fails to achieve an end goal, it may be because the theory was faulty, treatment was not provided at the appropriate level of intensity, or key intermediate objectives were not attained. In the example cited above, the finding that many clients maintained on methadone continued to commit crimes forced a reevaluation of the theory underlying

methadone treatment regarding the events which control criminal behavior. If the program which attempts to change several mediating variables in order to reduce criminality fails to achieve that end goal, it can
investigate whether all intermediate objectives in fact were attained.
Conversely, research might show that end goals were achieved in the absence of change in presumably key mediating variables, e.g., that reductions in criminality were achieved without changes in self-esteem. In
that case, intermediate objectives thought to be essential to the process
may be determined to be superfluous.

Generating a process description requires defining what the program
does, selecting or designing measures of the degree of implementation of
treatment elements, and gathering the data. There are several ways of
finding out what a program does: directly observing staff and clients;
talking with administrative and clinical staff about program activities;
talking with clients about what they do; reading the "official" program
description of the treatment regimen; and reading clinical files for
descriptions of individual treatment plans and recorded activities. Once
the treatment elements have been identified, measures of implementation appropriate to those elements must be selected. As mentioned
above, few measures of process elements exist which can be adopted or
adapted for use. However, Sechrest and Redner (1979) suggest some parameters for assessing treatment strength: amount of treatment per unit
of time, e.g., hours of group, individual, family, etc. counseling per
week; size of the group; extent of participation of staff and clients, e.g.,
how much people talk and what they talk about; duration of treatment;
qualifications of staff; and clarity of the treatment plan. If applicable,
one would also want to determine the type, quantity, and frequency of
the medications prescribed. Data sources may include a mix of direct
observation, staff and client self-report, and program records. Independent observers can estimate the amount of time which clients spend in
various activities as well as the types and frequency of behaviors they
enact. Checklists and questionnaires can be administered to staff and
clients to measure commitment to and satisfaction with treatment, as
well as perceived frequency, duration, and efficacy of treatment elements. Client records can be examined to determine whether a treatment plan exists, how detailed it is, and the extent to which it has been
followed.

When a program consists of one group counseling session a week a
process description is not very difficult, although the way in which the

counseling is provided needs to be documented. Describing the process of a residential program which provides 24-hour care seven days a week is much harder. "Treatment" in these programs may be so complex that one cannot easily determine where it starts and stops, much less measure it.

Treatment Process in TCs

Process variables in residential programs may be divided into three categories: 1) treatment "services" and other scheduled activities, such as group counseling and housekeeping assignments; 2) other change-induction structures, such as explicit schedules of rewards and sanctions; and 3) change-inducing behaviors.

a. **"Services" and other Scheduled Activities**. Many questions about treatment effectiveness are phrased in terms of service elements. For example, one might ask whether family therapy in conjunction with individual and group counseling is more effective in reducing drug use among adolescents than individual and group counseling alone. These treatment elements are also the easiest process variables to identify. They tend to be staff-led and offered in time-limited units. Program descriptions usually identify the services they provide. They also tend to be specified in treatment plans, so that one can compare the planned treatment to the treatment actually received. A checklist of 26 services which programs might offer is contained in the NIDA NDATUS (1983).

Residents also spend time in scheduled activities not traditionally classified as treatment services but which the program believes effect change. Such activities include unpaid facility tasks, ranging from cooking to fund-raising; paid jobs or school; and seminars and meetings which may be didactic or focus on skills training of various sorts. An on-site observer can readily determine whether or not these activities take place, and their frequency and duration. Information about other parameters of treatment strength, such as the nature and level of participation in counseling sessions, is obtainable with greater efforts.

We found it useful to group scheduled activities and services into five classes: 1) "treatment" activites, including individual, group, family, and other forms of counseling; 2) "functional" activities, including work assignments in the facility, "department" meetings, and household management skills training; 3) "productive" activities, such as paid employment outside the facility, degree and non-degree educational programs; 4) "reentry" activities, including vocational rehabilitation, job-seeking skills training, job counseling and placement, financial skills training, and training in the use of community resources; and 5) interpersonal activities, such as recreation and social skills training. Calculating the percentage of total scheduled time per week that residents spend in these different classes of activities provides a simple but useful summary of program activity.

b. **Other Change-Induction Structures**. Change induction structures and services overlap considerably, since services subsume events such as reinforcement and modeling presumed to facilitate change. In addition, however, the services take place in a social environment which itself can be structured to facilitate change, thus extending the concept of "treatment" from the traditional patient-therapist dyad, or even the group, to the community itself. These activities are not necessarily staff-directed or offered in measurable units of time, and they are not listed in an individual's treatment plan. Some examples of structures which residential programs make use of are hierarchical job structure, rewards and sanctions, role models and scripted verbal performances (Hawkins and Wacker, 1983).

Many residental programs encourage or require residents to perform chores around the house. These tasks can be distinguished from paid jobs and from vocational rehabilitation, where residents receive training in technical skills which are directly transferable to jobs in the greater community. Facility work assignments may range from light housekeeping to running the house. Programs' goals in involving residents in facilty work may range from trying to keep them occupied when they are not involved in other activities to trying to achieve a variety of cognitive, emotional, and behavioral changes. The intermediate objectives most commonly cited by programs that use work assignments to effect change include inculcating good work habits, such as showing up on time and taking directions; increasing tolerance to stress and learning how to work under pressure; learning problem-solving skills; learning to accept responsibility for others' welfare; increasing self-esteem through positive achievements; and integrating pro-social values, specifically, the value of "productive" work.

Some parameters for estimating whether work assignments are provided in a weak or strong form include: the tasks are voluntary or required; the tasks are "make work," as when the resident who sweeps the floor is followed by a paid janitor who "really" sweeps the floor, or the tasks are essential to the funtioning of the facility; the amount of time residents spend working; whether all tasks are of equal difficulty or are arranged hierarchically with respect to difficulty and responsibility; whether or not there is a "job description" specifying what the job entails and criteria for evaluating satisfactory performance; whether or not staff members are assigned to oversee departments; whether or not clients express pride in their work and associate increases in status and responsibility with advances up the job hierarchy, if one exists.

Programs sometimes designate certain activities as privileges, such as telephoning or weekend passes, to be earned with good behavior. They also can make use of sanctions to be levied for inappropriate behavior, ranging from a mild oral rebuke to explusion from the program. In general, the privileges and sanctions are tangible, physical events which can be distinguished from reinforcers such as the status and esteem the resident experiences from job promotions; other social reinforcers, such as attention, approval and affection; or the self-reinforcing feed-back the resident experiences by successfully completing a task. The effectiveness of these reinforcers to bring behavior into conformity with the standards of the community hypothetically can be increased by withholding the privileges for some period of time following admission. This serves to cut the resident off from his or her pretreatment environment (i.e., creates a state of deprivation) and makes the resident more dependent on the program's rewards.

Physical reinforcers, more so than social reinforcers, make the link between behavior and consequences very obvious. The rationale for employing such reinforcers is that some drug abusers do not associate their behavior and the consequences contingent upon that behavior. Either because consequences were never administered systematically in that person's lifetime or because the abuser has learned to defend against awareness of those consequences. Thus, the objective in using schedules of privileges and sanctions is not merely to shape particular behaviors, but to increase the resident's awarenss of and responsivity to the social environment. In essence what is being shaped is the resident's capacity to be reinforced by feedback from the environment.

In addition to describing the events designated by the program as privileges and sanctions, if any, the strength of this treatment element can be specified by means of the following parameters: how much time typically elapses before the privilege is granted; whether behavioral criteria for granting a privilege or levying a sanction are spelled out; the frequency of use of each event; the extent to which consequence are provided immediately or are delayed; the size of the unit of behavior which the community discriminates and reinforces, from very small (e.g., leaving a cigarette in an ashtray) to very large (e.g., remaining drug free for one year); and to what extent residents report that they work for privileges, try to avoid sanctions, and believe that they are helpful.

In general, modeling refers to the acquisition of new behaviors through the observation and imitation of the behaviors of others. Modeling in treatment settings can occur relatively informally, as when someone learns a new coping response by hearing another person describe how he or she dealt with a problem; or relatively formally, as when someone is required to reproduce a behavioral sequence which another person has demonstrated. In drug rehabilitation programs, staff and residents may also be expected to act as role models.

Programs will vary with respect to the degree to which residents are held responsible for achieving the community's goals. Programs may require only that residents work actively on their own problems. Others may expect residents to hold each other accountable for complying with treatment requirements as well as to be accountable for their own actions. Thus, being a "role model" may entail behaving according to community standards; or behaving appropriately as well as taking an active role in convincing others to do the same.

Many drug treatment programs employ ex-addicts as counselors. Some do so for purely economic reasons: ex-addict counselors typically are paid less than traditionally-trained counselors. Other programs may believe that ex-addict counselors are more effective with certain types of drug abusers than traditionally-trained counselors. If so, the researcher would want to find out if the program believes that ex-addict counselors do different things, or do similar things differently, than traditionally-trained counselors. Such hypothesized differences in procedure, if they exist, should be observable.

We suggest that programs also differentially emphasize what the ex-addict staff member represents rather than what he or she does. The program's "teachings" may specify that ex-addict staff "have been where the resident has been," have "made it" despite great handicaps, and have made it owing to the help of programs such as the one the resident is in. Thus, the presence of ex-addict staff may be expected to increase mutual identification and cohesion, increase the resident's expectations for success, and increase the resident's belief in the efficacy of the treatment procedures. While ex-addict staff in and of themselves may not induce change, they may increase the likelihood that residents will comply with treatment procedures which in turn should increase the likelihood of change.

In this section we are using "modeling" to refer to programs' **expectations** about how staff and residents should behave, on the assumption that differences in expectations will be associated with differences in the observed frequency of expected behaviors. In the next section we shall discuss the need to observe the extent to which staff and residents actually perform the expected behaviors. One may attempt to estimate differential emphasis on modeling by asking program staff whether being a good role model is a criterion for evaluating residents' progress; if the program employs ex-addict staff, what importance the program attaches to staff's recovered status, if any; and to what extent the program expects residents to hold each other accountable as well as to be supportive. If the effectiveness of ex-addict staff is presumed to be mediated by client expectancies, measures of these expectancies should be obtained. This could be in the form of a series of statements with which residents agree or disagree, such as staff have had experiences similar to those of residents, staff represent the possibility of change, the program can help residents to change, and the like.

Much of what is learned in treatment comes under the heading of verbal behavior. Clients learn new ways of talking about themselves and others by means of suggestion, modeling, differential reinforcement, and the like. Changes in the frequency, form and content of verbal expressions are assumed to be accompanied by cognitive changes, such as restructuring one's experience and adopting new ways of thinking about oneself and the world. The anticipated changes in verbal behavior and cognitions are guided by theories implicit in the treatment about what is effective in helping people achieve relief and solve problems. The emphasis on verbal expressiveness itself reflects assumptions about the relative efficacy of this particular activity as a means of solving problems.

Some drug treatment programs go beyond modeling verbal responses to what might be called "scripting." The phenomenon has been described at length by Hawkins and Wacker (1983) and Antze (1979). Briefly, scripts are chunks of verbal behavior which have been prescribed by the program as to approximate form, content and world view, although not necessarily to precise lines of dialogue. Scripted performances might be extemporaneous except for the great similarity they bear to one another. They usually are transmitted from staff to resident and from resident to resident orally rather than in writing. Some examples of scripted performances include describing the structure, function and rationale of the program; personal narratives, or telling one's life story recast according to the group's value system; confessions; confrontations, including pullups, haircuts and encounter groups; and the explanations that residents provide about what they did to earn a learning experience and what they are supposed to learn from experience.

Hypothetically, scripts are an efficient means of simultaneously achieving multiple goals. First, they teach communication skills. The scripts provide opportunities to practice verbal expressiveness to inarticulate residents or residents with little experience in verbalizing thoughts and feelings. Second, residents learn cognitive strategies for identifying and dealing with events which control drug use. The personal narratives often contain statements about why the person used drugs and what he or she must do to remain drug free. These self-statements may serve to remind the resident to enact the appropriate behavior in a problematic situation. Third, the scripts which govern the expression of negative, especially hostile feelings — pullups, haircuts, and other confrontations — not only teach residents how to express these emotions but also that there is a time and a place to do so. Thus, impulsive, acting-out behaviors are put under the control of the scripted situation. Finally, the scripts carry the program's ideology. By continually explaining the program's rationale to new admissions or describing how the program is helping him to change, a resident may end up internalizing the values he is expressing.

The researcher should be able to find out from staff and residents the extent to which verbal preformances are emphasized in treatment by means of questions such as: is there a program "philosophy," are residents expected to know the program "philosophy"; are residents expected to "tell their story" to each other and to visitors; do staff "structure" haircuts with respect to intensity and duration; are there different types of confrontations, from "light-weight" to a "blow-out"; are residents expected to report "inappropriate" verbal behavior to staff; is "talking about feelings" a measure of progress in treatment?

c. **Change-Inducing Behaviors.** Throughout this section on process we have been discussing the need to obtain measures of staff and client behaviors in describing treatment implementation. For example, clients' attendance records, how much they talk and what they talk about were suggested as measures of the strength of treatment services such as counseling. Similarly, clients' ratings of staff, such as their perceived similarity to residents and special understanding of residents' problems, were suggested as measures of the emphasis on modeling as a change-induction structure. While services subsume change-induction structures and both subsume behaviors, it is also possible to study behaviors themselves as treatment inputs. The frequency, intensity and content of interactions among residents will vary among programs and may be differentially associated with out come. It has been suggested, for example, that marginally-adjusted clients do better in programs where the frequency and intensity of interactions is low (Moos and Finney, 1983; Sechrest and Redner, 1979). Programs will also vary with respect to the importance placed on staff-to-resident versus resident-to-resident interactions.

The researcher who wishes to study behaviors must decide, at the very least, who does the observing and who and what is observed. A non-participant observer can record staff's behavior, residents' behavior, staff-with-resident interactions and resident-with-resident interactions. Staff and residents can record their perceptions of their own and others' behavior. There is a vast literature on psychotherapy (e.g., Orlinsky and Howard, 1978) and group processes (e.g., Yalom, 1975) which may help the researcher identify what aspects of behavior to measure. Or the researcher can generate a checklist by asking the program to describe what staff and residents do to facilitate change.

The Community-Oriented Programs Environment Scale (COPES) (Moos, 1974) records residents' general perceptions of resident and staff behaviors (there is also a staff form). In a true-false format, residents indicate whether people in the program express feelings, including negative ones; are supportive of one another; encourage independent problem solving; encourage mutual involvement; and the like. Levy (1979) identified 28 "help-giving" activities in groups such as behavioral prescription (i.e., "do this"), behavioral proscription (i.e., "don't do this"), behavioral rehearsal, positive reinforcement, punishment, modeling, self-disclosure, confrontation, and the like. Levy's items can be used as the basis of a self-report questionnaire or an observation instrument.

PRELIMINARY VALIDATION

We have conducted a preliminary evaluation of the ability of the suggested treatment variables to distinguish among programs. The study was concerned with describing and differentiating residential drug free (RDF) treatment programs classified as short-term (planned duration of treatment less than six months), middle-term (planned duration between six and 11 months), and long-term (planned duration 12 months or more). Survey data were obtained from 93 RDF programs. Archival data were obtained from the National Institute on Drug Abuse NDA-TUS and CODAP systems for 272 RDF programs, but will not be reported in detail here.

Short-term, middle-term, and long-term RDF programs differ with respect to organizational variables, the nature of the client population, and the nature of the treatment process.

Hierarchical Multiple Regression Analysis

A regression model was constructed to summarize the relationships among the three classes of predictor variables (organizational, client and process variables) and the dependent variable (planned duration of treatment for short, medium and long term programs). The classes of variables were entered into the equation in an order which reflects our assumptions about program management: irrespective of treatment philosophy, you must first have providers of treatment and financial support, then someone to treat, before you can begin treatment.

The five structural characteristics entered in the first step include primary orientation, physical environment, size of the client population (static population), number of full-time staff, and cost per client per day. The primary orientation categories were coded as follows: 1 = alcoholism services; 2 = drug and alcoholism services, and 3 = drug abuse services. Physical environment was coded dichotomously: 1 = hospital setting, 2 = non-hospital.

The seven client variables entered in the second step are the demographic characteristics of clients in treatment as of September 30, 1980. These include percent non-white, percent 20 and younger, percent 21 to 30, percent 31 and older, percent whose primary drug is a narcotic, percent whose primary drug is marijuana, and percent whose primary drug is alcohol.

The 16 process variables entered in the third step include the hours per week during the residential phase that residents spend in treatment, "functional," productive, reentry, and interpersonal activities (five variables); scale scores for the two privileges factors, the four sanctions factors, and the four client behaviors factors; and the rating of residents' responsibility for each others' treatment (see Holland, 1982, for details about scale scores).

The entire model accounts for 80 percent of the variance in planned duration (66% after adjusting for the number of variables in the equation).

The organizational variables account for 39 percent of total explained variance. Primary orientation alone accounts for 18 percent. Client characteristics add 15 percent to the explained variance, while the process variables account for the final 46 percent. It is of particular interest that the process variables add significantly to the model even when program and client variables are taken into account.

The variables with the highest correlations with duration of treatment include time spent in "functional" activities ($r = .56$); percentage of alcohol abusers in the client population ($r = -.49$); percentage of narcotics abusers in the client population ($r = .48$); primary orientation ($r = .42$); the first santions sub-scale ($r = .41$); the second privileges sub-scale ($r = .39$); the fourth behavioral sub-scale ($r = .39$); the second santions sub-scale ($r = .37$); the percentage of clients age 31 and older ($r = .37$); physical environment ($r = .34$); cost per client per day ($r = -.34$); and the amount of time spent in reentry activities ($r = .32$). Overall, though preliminary, these results support the validity of the framework proposed and in particular the relevance or the identified variables for measuring the treatment process in therapeutic communities.

Other investigators have made significant progress in explicating the treatment process of residential programs, including Moos and Finney (1983), Hawkins and Wacker (1983), and Sugarman (in this volumn). In this chapter we have presented what we believe is a fairly comprehensive list of process variables for residential programs. The purpose of this list is not to enumerate the features of the "ideal" or prototypical residential program. Rather, by developing a checklist of what residential programs might do, we hope to make the job of documenting the actual pattern and level of program activity a little easier. We also hope to encourage some consistency in observations across programs, thus facilitating comparative research.

Part III

THE FUTURE: ISSUES AND APPLICATION

CHAPTER 15

THE THERAPEUTIC COMMUNITY: LOOKING AHEAD

GEORGE DE LEON

THE TC IS AN experiment twenty years in progress. Despite vicissitudes of economic cycles, swings in society's perception of drug abuse and shifts in public policy, the TC has survived. Though still evolving, it has established itself as a significant alternative approach to the treatment of drug abuse. This paper explores several broader considerations concerning the future of TCs.

The TC, Mental Health and Substance Abuse

For a variety of reasons, the drug abuse client in treatment has not attracted the respect, interest or involvement of the mental health establishment. Nevertheless, the pressure has mounted on mental health institutions to identify and treat a growing substance abuse problem among psychiatric patient populations. This has increased their receptivity to TC models albeit in modified formats.

Extensive use of the substances by inpatient psychiatric patients is commonly reported by staff and is currently being documented. In particular, among young adults in mental hospitals (young adult chronics), a substantial proportion of the inpatient population ages 18-35, drug use poses serious management and clinical problems. Although the cause and effect questions remain unresolved, there is little doubt that the availability and use of substances produces symptoms or exacerbates pre-existing psychiatric conditions.

Evidence also suggests that there is considerable substance use among the population of outpatient ambulatory clients whose undetected drug use and its contribution to the clinical picture of the individual's adjustment presents a formidable diagnostic problem. This has lately given rise to the need for a dual diagnostic category (e.g., psychiatric plus substance abuse) in assessing clients in outpatient settings.

The involvement of the mental health system in substance use represents both threat and opportunity to therapeutic communities. North American TCs have been wary of the mental health system for several reasons (see for example, De Leon & Beschner, 1977). For example, the mental health system is politically, fiscally and scientifically more well entrenched than the recently assembled drug treatment and research system. Many scientists, health care professionals, legislators and policy makers view drug misuse as variants of mental health problems. Mental health professionals still tend to explain the drug abuse problem in psychological-psychiatric jargon as do medical specialists in a biological vernacular. Similarly, they tend to ignore the advances accomplished by the main treatment modalities developed specifically for drug abuse. The unique approach to treating drug abuse problems in TCs is often retranslated into mental health concepts which can obscure its special character. This is particularly evident among the TCs within certain psychiatric settings, inpatient alcohol and short term V.A. programs.

Moreover, increasing numbers of mental health practitioners are involved in the substance abuse problem. These professionals have the social benefit of status and authority. Thus, their role in substance abuse could gradually supercede those of the paraprofessionals, most of whom have been recovered ex-addicts and who have been most effective in treating substance abuse problems.

The above threats also present a certain opportunity for the TC to consolidate its position, and further evolve as a health care institution. TCs have developed a powerful approach to successfully treating many drug abusers. To prevent the dilution of the model, the TC is currently attempting to codify its principles and practices. This explicit rendering of TC theory, practice and training could exert a positive influence on the mental health system itself. Rather than co-option, there is the real possiblity that the traditional human service establishment can be positively influenced by the TC.

Similarly, outpatient counseling centers serving larger numbers of families and adolescents with substance abuse problems have much to learn from the TC approach. Some TCs have developed outpatient modalities which appear to be successfully treating substance abusers based upon TC principles.

Finally, the current trends protend the development of a new TC model incorporating elements of the traditional TC approach, appropriate psychiatric techniques and established practices developed in the Jones therapeutic community model. Several writers have proposed that a common TC model could serve varieties of psychiatric and/or substance abuse clients (e.g., De Leon, 1983; Jones, 1980; Sugarman, this volumn).

A broader issue concerns the larger social community. The TC approach to individual change is fundamentally consistent with good parenting and self management. However, enculturation of recreational drug use has implicitly sanctioned substance use particularly among adolescents. In the present social climate of pervasive drug use, traditional TCs can play a unique role as service provider and educator. From the TC perspective, abstinence or moderation reveals self control and an increased capacity to tolerate the frustrations inherent in social and interpersonal pressures without recourse to quick relief or escape. This perspective can be translated to the larger community through drug prevention and early intervention efforts which reinforce values and conduct with respect to drug use.

This role function is depicted in two illustrations. Some TCs have been a resource for developing parent organizations against youth drug use in the U.S.A. The basic family surrogate approach in TCs resonates the attitudes and values of these groups.

Also, drug education and drug prevention projects have long been under way in several traditional TCs in North America. These, however, have not yet been empirically evaluated.

"Beware of Constantine"

The rate of evolutionary change in therapeutic communities toward an established human services institution has been notably rapid. This is particularly evident in review of change since January, 1976 when the first assembly of TC programs convened in Washington, D.C. (see De Leon & Beschner, 1977). Several of the main agenda items of that milestone meeting are now significant accomplishments.

First, the national organization of Therapeutic Communities of America (TCA) consisting of over 100 full and corresponding member therapeutic communities has firmly established its visibility and credibitlity as the voice of the drug free treatment approach and philosophy in the U.S.A. In a few short years, this organization has demonstrated effectiveness in influencing funding priorities, disseminating information throughout the field and strengthening the cohesiveness of the therapeutic community modality.

On a larger scale, there has emerged a World Federation of Therapeutic Communities (WFTC) represented by programs from all continents and many nations. This organization has sponsored seven world conferences and published five books of preceedings. It symbolizes the elaboration of the therapeutic community approach into a human services movement, evident in the rising number of regional therapeutic community organizations throughout the world.

Second, upgrading the skills and practices of therapeutic community workers has been advanced through an explicit credentialling process. The national organization (TCA) has established criteria and procedures for evaluating counselors and certifying their competency. This critical step paves the way toward strengthening the professionalization of addiction specialists.

Third, management, fiscal, administrative and research sophistication are now apparent in the therapeutic community modality. Most of larger and older programs incorporate the hardware and software of modern corporate organizations to facilitate operations and seek continued management education training. Some have developed program-based research and evaluation capability, others are participants in scientific efforts. Old issues of anti-intellectual bias have receded as is evident in the steady recruitment of workers from all specialties to provide ancillary services and to strengthen administrative operations.

These advances notwithstanding, a certain anxiety that pervaded the 1976 conferees lingers today. Then, fiscal survival compelled TCs to ambivalently accept institutionalization which for many portended a loss of identity. Now, ironically, its status as an established healthcare institution has mitigated its survival fears but not the possibility of oblivion through mutation.

Can the TC alternative, supported and nurtured by the establishment, thrive in its original form which presumably is the basis of its success? Currently, that question cannot be clearly answered.

The uniqueness and strength of the TC lay in it fundamental elements of self help and community as healer. Its original form, and perhaps its fate resemble those of its historical prototypes. These quasi-religious groupings spontaneously arose among the disaffiliated as responses to societies which failed to help and they disappeared often through assimilation.

Unlike its prototype, the 20th century TC is a hybrid spawned from a union of public support and self help. Thus, bureaucracy, accountability, professionalization and the increased distance from its first generation roots, are factors which could radically change the self help character of the TC. While these institutional attributes can assure its survival, they could pollute its humanistic ecology and devitalize its community dynamic.

Nevertheless, this phase of the TC experiment may yet prove to the be the most exciting. Its essential "curative" elements, community, self help, individual commitment, role modeling and social learning may be transmittable forces mediated more through the attitude, conduct, values and vision of the people involved in the process rather than its institutional framework. Thus, the TC can remain immune from the potentially dehumanizing influences of technology, professionalization, management and bureaucracy by utilizing the advantages of these in the service of its purpose, the positive transformation of human lives.

CHAPTER 16

USES AND ABUSES OF POWER AND AUTHORITY WITHIN THE AMERICAN SELF-HELP RESIDENTIAL THERAPEUTIC COMMUNITY: A PERVERSION OR A NECESSITY?

THOMAS E. BRATTER
EDWARD P. BRATTER
JESSICA F. HEIMBERG

THE AMERICAN residential self-help therapeutic community needs to codify and simultaneously evaluate the positive and noxious impacts of the utilization of power. This inquiry is not concerned with documenting the numerous specific examples of the abuse of power known to the insiders but, instead, prefers to attempt to present an overview so those who are more passionately involved with therapeutic communities will begin to discuss these issues. While some surely will respond defensively to a perceived criticism, the intent of this chapter is a warning because unless some checks and balances are implemented without delay, the debacle which characterized Synanon may not be an isolated phenomenon but can threaten the entire American residential self-help therapeutic community movement. It is sobering to read the candid and graphic accounts of Anson (1978), Deitch & Zweben (1979), and Mitchel, Mitchel & Ofshe (1980) who describe the problems which beset Synanon. More recently, Weppner (1983) discusses the disgrace and demise of Matrix House, a third generation therapeutic community, funded by the National Institute of Mental Health which was housed in the Federal Penitentiary at Lexington, Kentucky. The number of charismatic leaders who directed therapeutic communities to greatness only to become consumed by their abuse of power tragically continues to proliferate. No longer can the American self-help therapeutic community afford either to ignore or to deny this disquieting reality of the mismanagement of power. There are cracks in the basic structure that need repair to ensure survival of a most innovative and pragmatic quasi-commune, quasi-treatment approach which is too valuable to be consumed by the quest for personal power.

Mowrer (1977) believes that the 19th century religious and utopian communes were the spiritual progenitors of the TC. A descendant of the Oneida Community, Robertson (1970) has provided a most illuminating autobiography. Yablonsky (1962 & 1965) and Casriel (1963) have credited Dederich with being the genius behind Synanon. The creator of Synanon was conversant with the literature discussing the Oneida Community and with the writings of Emerson (1803-1882) (1913) and Thoreau (1817-1862) (1899) both of whom were among the most influential American Transcendental philosophers of the 19th century.

Bassin (Shelly & Bassin, 1964 & 1965) wrote the grant for the original Daytop Lodge, the precursor to Daytop Village, had parents who lived in the Clarion (Utah) commune. These communes, at the very least were a spirtual ancestor to the TC, were created by those individuals whose values and beliefs conflicted with those of the larger society and who sought to create their own utopian self-sufficient communities, were chronicled by Hinds (1878), Harvey (1949), Sarns (1959), Royer, (1966), Carden (1969) and Roberts (1971).

Why is there any need to study power and authority in the American self-help therapeutic community? Simply stated, if the residential TC wishes to prevail as a dominant force in the 21st century, clearly it must possess the courage of its convictions while maintaining its integrity to examine the abuses of power and in so doing, find corrective solutions, or, like the 19th century commune movement which neglected to maintain the delicate balance between freedom and power, may be relegated to another interesting, but transitory, experiment in residential living. Freudenberger (1974), Rachman (1974), Bratter (1978) and Horn (1978) have warned about abuses of power within the self-help therapeutic community. Unless, therefore, power can be used constructively and creatively, the TC will become extinct.

Power and Authority: Curative or Noxious?

If it were possible to reduce the history of civilization to two dependent variables, the salient issues would be: (1) the use and abuse of power and (2) the society's individual and collective relationship to authority. Power, authority, and influence (either their presence or their absence) are intrinsic to any social organization whether it is democratic or totalitarian. Power is indispensable in both the macrocosmic society and the microcosmic community because without it, there would be anarchy. Tonnies (1957) has contributed a significant treatise discussing the relationship between geminschaft (community) and gesellschaft (society). The concept of power needs to be understood because the potential for exploitation of the weaker is obvious. Power is required, however, to control the behavior of the masses. Weber (1947), in fact, describes valid forms of power which can be justified when three conditions are fulfilled:

1. **Rational ground** — resting on a belief in the "legality" of patterns of normative rules and the right of those elevated to authority under such rules to issue commands.
2. **Traditional grounds** — resting on an established belief in the sanctity of immemorial traditions and the legitimacy of the status of those exercising authority under them (traditional authority).
3. **Charismatic grounds** — resting on devotion to the specific and the exceptional sanctity; heroism or exemplary character of an individual person, and of the normative patterns of order revealed or ordained by him (charismatic authority).

Power is neither an asset nor a liability but instead, depends upon how it is administered and for what purpose(s). Those in power can increase/decrease compensation and freedom, can determine punishments, penalties and/or provide promotions/commendations. The powerful can influence the quality of life for their subordinates. The delicate balance between the needs of society and those of the individual needs constant scrutiny. Recognizing that effective leaders must be sensitive to the potential conflict between the democratic goals of the microcosm and the autocratic goals of the macrocosm, Wolberg (1975) believes that responsible leaders must help others achieve this kind of awarness. "He must become an activist on social and political levels as well as on personal . . . informing the public as to ways in which its democratic preference are sacrificed to the perpetuation of the aggressive power of larger societal structures." Bentham (1914) formulated his basic principle of Utilitarianism which constitutes the basis for many social philosophies:

> The science of legislation consists, therefore, in determining what makes for the good of the particular community whose interests are at stake, while its

art consists in contriving some means of realization. . . Three conditions
must be fulfilled:

First, we must attach to the word Utility, a clear and precise connotation.

. .

Second, we must assert the supreme and undivided sovereignty of this
principle by rigorously discarding each other. . . No exception to its applicability can, in any circumstances, be allowed.

Thirdly, we must discover some calculus or process of "moral arithmetic"
by means of which we may arrive at uniform results. . . Nature has placed
mankind under the governance of two sovereign masters, Pleasure and Pain.

The American therapeutic community utilizes a relatively simplisitic
behavioral paradigm. For those who refuse to conform and who disobey
the mandate, there will be a series of punishments. For those, however,
who produce and behave responsibility, they are rewarded by being promoted and being given more status. There exists a fluid upward
dynamic. In the military, for example, rank readily is discerned by the
number of stripes or the insignia worn on the uniform. In the TC, however, in comparison, status is determined by the number of privileges
the individual gains. Sleeping quarters, amount of leisure time, number
of individuals who report directly to the person, etc., are indicative of
status. Status is allocated by those who are in power to demostrate
tangibly how they believe the residents is progressing. These types of
evaluations, based essentially on productivity and attitude, serve as an
incentive to improve one's self because the awarding of tangible privileges combine to make existence within a TC more pleasurable. When
either the resident or a staff member is guilty of "deviant" or dysfunctional behavior, privileges and rank can be decreased. Unacceptable behavior has immediate consequences which can serve as a learning
experience for those who commit any infraction. Simultaneously with
any demotion is a specific explanation which describes the undesirable
behavior plus instruction not only how to avoid this type of situation but
also what specifically can be done to rectify the incident in an effort to
regain privileges. Power in the TC is both horizontal and vertical. Both
the staff and the residents will be promoted or demoted solely on the basis of their behavioral performance. The social structure of the residential program involves an elaborate hierarchy which contains within it a
strict system of rewards and punishments. Much of the controversy,
rightfully so, is especially generated by those who are outside the TC
movement. This produces a galvanizing gulf of communication associated precisely with the use and abuse of power by charismatic leaders
as it relates both to individual and institutional change.

There is reason to believe that Jones (1952, 1953, 1968, & 1976), a psychiatrist, who attempted to humanize mental institutions by creating a professional model of the therapeutic community which predates the self-help concept by a decade, agrees with Rosseau. Working with a hospitalized subpopulation, Jones remains idealistic and positive about patients' desires about improving themselves while concurrently ridding themselves of symptoms. Rubel, Bratter, Smirnoff, Thompson & Baker (1982) have documented the fundamental differences between the Jones's model and that of the self-help movement even though Jones (1979) attempts to argue both are similar by using reductionist thinking and a priori logic. Jones's ideas about the validity of democracy in mental institutions which are administered by credentialled physicians, in comparison to recovered persons, makes sense. Another inherent difference between the American self-help therapeutic community and the Jones's model is the notable lack of psychopathology and deceit of the patients. There exists a more pronounced barrier because credentialled professionals have been trained to treat symptomology of patients rather than to identify with them. The most startling distinction between the professional therapeutic model which has been developed by Jones and the American Self-Help TC is the utilization and reliance on recovered persons, as Bratter (1977a, b & 1980) reports, who become the primary treatment agents. In contrast to credentialled professionals who have been trained to treat symptomology, recovered persons function as responsible role models. Deitch (1983) writes, "With respect to role models, the presence of former addicts who have 'made it' is a crucial ingredient in the treatment method, supplying in the process of struggle, a concrete stimulus for hope to the client." Residents are encouraged to seek out a staff person and form a quasi-treatment, quasi-friendship based on the principles of trust, affection, and identification. As the resident discusses personal concerns with the staff member, the recovered person identifies with either the expressed or unconscious feelings by offering pragmatic solutions and suggestions. In direct proportion to the resident's stability and personal growth, the demarkation of authority boundaries dissolve until a relationship of equality is formed. Subtly, but systematically, the resident seeks to emulate the responsible role model. This process incorporates the psychoanalytic concepts of introjection, and identification. The residents wishes to gain the approbation, respect, trust, and friendship of the staff member. In a very real sense, the healthy family dynamic is created whereby initial dependence is de-

creased to the point of independence and actualized as the level of functioning between the two individuals becomes more similar and the reduction of the social barrier is effectuated.

Psycho-Social Characteristics of Drug-Dependents: Their Nihilism and Need to Believe in a Person More Powerful Than Themselves

Psychotropic prescriptions permit pleasure seekers to escape from a
reality they judge to be too pathetic, too painful, and too pessimistic to
endure. This conscious choice to self-mediate produces an insidious res-
ignation that enables addicted persons to conclude they have been excluded from any positive and productive place in the educational and
business environment. Alcoholically and drug addicted individuals un-
wittingly have trapped themselves in a "no win" — "no exit" labyrinth
where the only negative self-fulfilling prophesy is continued failure.
Substance abusers, who have been labelled by others, accept those acri-
monious assessments for themselves. Addicts have been told they are
uneducable, untreatable, untamed, unreliable, unwanted and unloved.
Addicts have significant deficits — they lack motivation, strength, ambition, and integrity because they avoid personal responsibility by remaining dishonest. Psychoanalytically, addicts have been portrayed as
having weak ego structures, defective superegos, inadequate psychosex-
ual development which produce pathological personal identities. They
fear success. They refuse to accept any responsibility. Pharmacological
pleasure seekers, furthermore, have a low threshold for any sort of physical or psychological pain such as personal criticism and rejection.
Whenever substance abusers experience fear, frustration, and failure,
they rely on instantaneous, superficial and ephemeral chemical cop-outs
rather than seeking contructive and creative solutions. Not surprisingly,
addicts remain intransigent about discontinuing their drug dependence
because they adamantly believe it is the only guaranteed concurrent activity which not only can achieve temporary relief from suffering but
also can produce pleasurable peace.

By definition, addicts suffer from monomania because they are pre-
occupied with securing drugs which will provide immediate gratification
from their pain. Substance abusers will consider any plan, no matter
how unrealistic, sadistic, and dangerous, to secure drugs. Social contacts are confined to those who are members of the same drug-related
fraternity or sorority. Addicted individuals become alienated from their
families and their friends and in advanced stages, even from themselves.

By virtue of their continual manipulation, deceit, and illicit behavior, drug dependents are trusted by no one. They are isolated, lonely and lost because they systematically have eliminmated social contacts in their perpectual pursuit of potent pharmacological substances. Addicts are depressed, demoralized, and desperate. They have ceased to dream. They no longer dare to believe in their potential to achieve happiness and success. They no longer know how to justify to themselves their existences. They are brusied, battered, beaten. Addicts simply have stopped believing in anyone or anything other than drugs to be the magic elixir for the agony of their pitiful existence.

Many Europeans and psychoanalysts believe addicted character-disordered persons are motivated to become abstinent with a minimum amount of therapeutic intervention. Zimmer-Hofler & Widmer (1981) reflect this attitude when they report, "What is astonishing is that 144 of 156 clients are motivated to renounce drugs," so they condemn the treatment approach of the American self-help program:

> In the sixties the almost imperialistic wave of the new TC flooded the USA and swamped the Europe. Horror-stories of bald heads, drastic punishments, rigid accusations, people being pilloried, self-accusations, aggressive group-confrontations and uncompromising hierarchy in a big subculture called Synanon reached us.

> Was it an archaic break into our civilization? Some were shocked and prone to ask for official prohibition of this new movement, even more since no trained psychotherapist was working at Synanon. An Ex-Alcoholic had succeeded in attracting addicts in troops, motivated to renounce drugs under the roughest conditions. From intellectuals down to the worst criminals, heroin addicts came to submit without condition and made from hard confrontations a new philosophy.

The critics of the self-help TCs object to the pragmatic emphasis on the acquisition of vocational and educational skills which they equate with some sort of political brain-washing. Programs in Europe, for example, tend to be more existential; which stresses personal freedom. Both Europeans and psychoanalysts appear to confuse the deliberate structural rigidity which is the treatment "sine qua non" when treating addicts with sadistic and countertherapeutic behavior. Sugarman (1974) explicitly has provided the treatment rational for the self-help TC:

> . . . based on the assumption that drug addicts have never grown up in terms of emotional and moral development. Thus the function of Daytop is to give residents a second chance to grow up in this sense. Their period of residency is recapitulation of their lost years. They are required to live under a regime of restrictions more appropriate to children or infants than to adults. And the rules under which they live are stated in absolute, harsh,

black-and-white terms in much the same way as young children interpret the rules of society to be. Indeed, the Daytop moral system is perhaps more rigidly fundamentalist than that of early childhood, for it is being used to teach a sense of values to people who have (unlike the young child) already acquired a warped sense of values. . . The ethical fundamentalism of Daytop has other qualities besides the harsh rigors. . . One of these elements, sometimes labelled "the Protestant Ethic," may be defined as the notion that many should strive to overcome any obstacles to his ambition. . . To resign oneself to accept hardships or difficulties is held to be dishonorable whereas to struggle to overcome them is praiseworthy. . . This ethic is a central feature of North American culture [which is misunderstood] in a narrow and materialistic sense.

Both the European professionals and psychoanalysts believe essentially that a "laissez faire leader" who has been discussed by Lippett & White (1952) can be an effective catalyst. This thinking is reminiscent of Locke who believed that government did need much power to regulate abuses and prohibit acts which conflict with the common good because individuals fundamentally are decent and respectful of others. In contrast to this optimistic and unrealistic view, the American self-help movement, which has been summarized cogently by Iverson & Wenger (1978), portray, drug dependents as "basically immature and irresponsible, and consequently have made stupid decisions in the past — they must, therefore, be given an opportunity to mature and to learn to accept responsibility." It becomes precisely this difference which has produced confusion and condemnation by both the Europeans and psychoanalysts regarding what works most effectively for addicted individuals.

The Charismatic Leader: A Study of Positive Leadership Qualities

During the last two decades of the twentieth century, society has seen the demise of the nuclear family whose security has been undermined by extra-marital affairs, desertions, divorces, and deaths. Families are continually uprooted geographically because individuals look for more lucrative jobs to help combat inflation. Alienation and loneliness become pervasive realities. It is no wonder that individuals are vulnerable and want to find a sense of commuity so they can feel as if they belong. The search for the benign, but benevolent, leader who can offer some degree of protection and caring continues from childhood until death. This quest to locate the individual who embodies these qualities for drug-dependents may be greater for some than for others because they have lost their ability to believe in someone else and have any faith about the inherent goodness of people.

The American self-help TC believes what depressed, despondent, self-destructive drug-dependents desperately need are charismatic and caring persons who can function as gurus and/or medicine men. These charismatic leaders assume the primary functions of the shaman, described by Kiev (1964), who restore hope, maintain high expectations for improvement, and instill faith of the individual-in-distress in the designated leader. Orne (1968) recognized the critical aspect of the healing relationship can begin when individuals feel: (1) That his problem can be potentially relieved. . . (2) That effective means of bringing about the desired change exist. . . and (3) That the therapist (is) willing and able to provide the means by which the desired changes may take place. Frank (1961), who has studied the relationship of persuasion and healing, has noted that the restoration of faith in one's ability to succeed is the crucial element in all forms of psychotherapy. It is this quasi-magical, quasi-mysterious charismatic quality which may be required to motivate addicts to begin to want to consider reclaiming their lives from chemical oblivion. It is impossible to impute the therapeutic value when a powerful, respected, and charismatic person exudes confidence and optimism that remission, rehabilitation, and recovery are realistic and, become the expected treatment outcomes. One way to accomplish this is to have programs which are managed by recovered persons who are responsible role models demonstrating that sobriety is possible. These charismatic leaders, in addition to being inspirational, are living proof that constructive and creative change is possible.

The single most important characteristic is a strong authority figure who can work with devious and psychopathological individuals. Ruocco (1981) not only has described the virtues of the charismatic leader who he calls a "benevolent dictator" but also provides the treatment rationale:

> The "Benevolent Dictator" historically has been the most distinguished model to teach desirous behavior. . . It contains two of the most important ingredents that most human beings are responsive to — "Love and Authority." . . . In the absence of authority, love becomes over-indulgence, a smothering crippler of self-sufficiency. Also without the tempering effect of love, authority becomes tyranny. . . Love cannot be more important to a child's well-being than the consistant presence of authority figures in his life. Love provides meaning to his life, a reason to strive. Authority provides direction to his strivings. These are not to be viewed as opposites because they work best when used together. . . The "Benevolent Dictator" is a system which has succeeded at establishing a nurturing yet firmly authoritative relationship.

Significantly, what enables the American self-help residential programs to be relatively effective with character disordered addicted individuals is the reliance on the charismatic leader. With their misunderstanding and prohibition of the charismatic leader, no wonder that psychoanalysis has remained woefully ineffective with drug and alcoholically addicted individuals. Elsewhere, we (Bratter et al., 1985) have enumerated specific reasons why psychoanalysis has failed to become a viable treatment modality for character-disordered individuals, which falls outside the purview of this chapter. The positive personal magnetism initially literally is the force required to pull drug dependents from the quagmire of addiction. It is precisely this charisma which is the quintessential quality for those who wish to become the significant factor to help individuals extricate themselves from their self-imposed slavery. In this aspect, the American Self-Help TC borrows from Machiavelli who portrayed individuals as being stupid, irrational, incapable of controlling their lives, and unable to govern themselves. Machiavelli (1940) proposes that a strong sovereign is needed. "Those who have been present at any deliberative assemblies of men will have observed how erroneous their opinions are; and, in fact, unless they are directed by superior men, they are apt to be contrary to all reason." The sovereign, or prince, therefore, needs to employ force ruthlessly. "Whoever becomes the ruler of a free city and does not destroy it, can expect to be destroyed by it, for it can always find a motive for rebellion in the name of liberty and of its ancient usages." Recognizing that charismatic leadership can contribute positively to the recovery process, Galanter (1982) asks, "In what other contexts may further understanding of the psychology of charismatic large groups prove to be useful?" Galanter recognizes that the utilization of charismatic techniques can be salutary in many of the self-help programs which provide intensive services to alcoholically and drug addicted individuals.

Lieberman, Yalmon & Miles (1973) have described the charismatic leader as "one who . . . (is) inspiring, imposing, stimulating . . . (believes) in himself . . . (has) a strong sense of mission." By this definition, the charismatic person becomes the central force which possesses the power to energize the group. Charisma intrinsically is neither an asset nor a liability but depends on its intent and the end product. Christ (1975) posits that the charismatic leader "tends to create a group which is dependent on him, will see in his person the focus of their interaction, and will experience a feeling of support, release of tension, and freeing up of emotions." When working with drug dependents, in specific, as I have written (Bratter, 1985), initially, unless the group leader is willing to assume the awesome charismatic role, there will be no incentive to terminate all drug-related dysfunctional behavior. Charisma, when applied therapeutically and judiciously, can become a curative catalyst to produce a correctional emotional experience. Rutan & Rice (1981) concur, "The creation of a charismatic leader to rescue the members is a natural response. Our patients often come to us yearning for a perfect parent, an omnipotent leader, the 'right' answers for life's questions. A more difficult task in parenting our children is the capacity to allow them to grow separate and apart. It is also a difficult task in therapy we provide."

The Autocratic Leader: A Perversion of Power and Trust

While the charismatic leader is motivated by altruism with some narcisstic compensation, in contrast, the Draconian autocrat craves the acquisition of personal power for self-aggrandizement with no concern for the welfare of others under his/her rule. The American self-help TC has witnessed many examples when charismatic leaders have been consumed by their quest for personal power. Liff (1975) rightfully so protests the abuse of charismatic leaders, "I am concerned that these group leaders, in their eagerness to heal and cure, tend to violate the dignity as well as the privacy of the person — his right not to participate, to be quiet, to withdraw without ridicule, humiliation, reprisal, or rejection of the leader himself or of other group members." Kemp (1964) suggests that of the authoritarian leader, "assumes that his decisions are superior to that of the group and that he is responsible for influencing the group to accept his views and plans. To achieve this result, he may use questions, suggestions, commands, interpretation, analysis, clarification, acceptance, reflection . . . if necessary, he will reinforce his position by reward or punishment." Individual and program problems proliferate when leaders become intrusive, challenging, noxious, authoritarian which is exacerbated by the dictorial, distorted, and demonic thinking that "I alone know what is right and good. I am the Savior, the Supreme Being." Decisions are made to glorify the self with a concurrent negation of the validity of the contributions, insights and rights of others. Any disagreement, no matter how legitimate or constructive, becomes convoluted into a paranoic personal attack that demands harsh retribution and retaliation to the perpetrators. Such ruthless domination and exploitation can be characterized by a reign of terror and a fear of saying or doing the wrong thing which will displease the leader. Fromm (1941), furthermore, illuminates the power megalomania of the autocratic leader's attitude toward the acquistion of unmitigated personal power when he writes:

> For the authoritarian character, there exists . . . two sexes: the powerful ones and the powerless ones. . . Power fascinates him not for any values for which a specific power may stand, but just because it is power. Just as his "love" is automatically aroused by power, so powerless people or institutions automatically arouse his contempt. The very sight of a powerless person makes him want to attack, dominate, humiliate him.

This type of autocratic control has been observed in cults that sought to isolate themselves while simultaneously arming themselves. This malignant phenomenon infiltrated both Synanon and Matrix House. The Guayana Mass Suicide was orchestrated by a demonic spiritual leader who demanded to be adulated and obeyed by all. Lewis (1935) has created an admittedly fictionalized, but sobering account of the rise of absolute totalitarianism in America which he entitled, "It Can't Happen Here." How different are the circumstances, the personalities, the psychopathology between Jonestown and Synanon and Matrix House? The only difference, perhaps, may be the degree of absolute corruption of a malignantly proliferating personal quest for power and the refusal to be accountable to anyone. All the ingredients which produced a mass suicide of staggering proportions in all probability are incubating in every therapeutic community that can be ignited upon the emergence to power of the autocratic-demonic leader. Equally alarming is Fromm's (1955) pronouncement about various totalitarian governments because the specific mechanism he describes has been detected in may therapeutic communities:

> Facism, Nazism and Stalinism have in common that they offered the atomized individual a new refuge and security. These systems are the culmination of alienation. The individual is made to feel powerless and insignificant, but taught to project all his human powers into the figure of the leader, the state, the "fatherland," to whom he has to submit and whom he has to worship. He escapes from freedom into a new idolatry.

Rational Authority: An Essential Ingredient to Effective Leadership

De Leon is correct when he contends that:

> Drug abuse is a **disorder of the whole person**. Although individuals differ in choice of substance, socio-economic or cultural background, abuse involves

some or all areas of functioning. Cognitive, behavioral, and medical problems appear as do mood disturbances. Thinking may be unrealistic or disorganzied. Values are confused, non-existent or antisocial. . . And, whether couched in existential or psychological terms, moral, religious or even spiritual issues are apparent.

De Leon contends that the psychological and intellectual deficits of addicted individuals must be ameliorated before any recovery can occur. Initially, it is impossible to establish a treatment relationship based on equality. Inevitably, a superior authority will be interacting with the individual-in-distress. Recognizing this reality, Fromm has described a form of leadership as rational authority which refers to a specific interpersonal relationship where the person-in-distress relates to the helper as being in a more powerful authoritative position. Fromm (1955, 1973), however, compares rational authority appropriately to the teacher-student relationship:

> The more the student learns, the less wide is the gap between him and the teacher. He becomes more and more like the teacher. In other words, the rational authority relationship tends to dissolve itself. . . In the rational authority kind of authority, the strength of the emotional ties will tend to decrease in direct proportion to the degree in which the person subjected to the authority becomes stronger and thereby more similar to the authority.

The recovered person, who functions as the helper, can offer assistance based on previous common experiences plus a recently acquired awareness and competence, according to Brill & Lieberman (1969):

> In a favorable position to offer suggestions, criticism, and support and to serve as a conventional role model to help the addict recreate his life style along more favorable lines. . . In the sense of providing a firm structuring of the treatment relationship, setting limits, and providing controls through the use of a graduated series of sanctions, it was conjectured that rational authority might minimize the addict's acting-out behavior, help him grow within this structure and internalize the controls he lacks, and hopefully, help him give up his destructive way of life.

Rational authority, furthermore, simultaneously helps the deficient learn how to reorient their attitudes and restructure interpersonal relationships so they can exist within the social system. Rational authority initially is an advice-giving, learning-based quasi-psychotherapeutic quasi-educational leadership orientation that utilizes realistic confrontations and programmed learning experiences which are designed to correct distorted attitudes and dysfunctional behavior. De Leon (1983)

accurately assesses the ultimate treatment benefits of rational authority
when he writes:

> For the disaffiliated, rational authority can facilitate acquiring personal auton-
> omy. The client's dysfunction often stems from historical difficulties with
> authorities, parental or otherwise, who have not been trusted or perceived as
> guides and teachers. Autonomy (which involves self-authority) is most effec-
> tively learned through a positive experience with credible "other" authority fig-
> ures seen as supportive, correcting and protecting. Becoming one's own
> authority is mediated through a successful experience with rational authority.

Conclusion. Behavioral Control: Peril or Promise?

In all democratic societies and institutions, there is a perpetual delicate dynamic which needs constant monitoring and resolution betwen
the preservation of individual freedom versus the same subordination to
the power of those entrusted to leadership positions. Only anarchists
would refute the right which any democratic organization has to protect
itself from the abuses of those who violate the fundamental social contract. Kittrie (1971) acknowledges that the legal system protects the individual from governmental excesses but decries the lack of controls when
the State functions in the capacity of "Parens Patriae" and the "Therapeutic State." Skinner (Rogers & Skinner, 1956) discusses the problem of
the moral responsibility of scientists and philosophers who discuss control:

> The dangers inherent in the control of human behavior are very real. The
> possibility of misuse of scientific knowledge must always be faced. We can-
> not escape by denying the power of a science of behavior or arresting its de-
> velopment. It is no help to cling to familiar philosophies of human behavior
> simply because they are more reassuring. . . The new techniques emerging
> from a science of behavior must be subject to the explicit counter control
> which already has been applied to earlier and cruder forms.

Rogers (Rogers & Skinner, 1956) poses the primary philosophical and
moral issue regarding social and political control when he asks: "Who
will be controlled? Who will exercise control? What type of control will
be exercised? Most important of all, toward what end or what purpose,
in the pursuit of what values, will control be exercised?"

The residential American Self-Help Therapeutic Community must
remember that it needs to protect the individual's constitutional rights
and not violate them when the concepts of "treatment" become confused
with "social control." Shapiro (1972) provides important guidelines when
he advocates there needs to be:

> An explicit articulation of the specific goals. . . ; and a sensitive consider-

ation of the very difficult legal and moral issues at stake. These requirements necessitate a careful review of the major concepts that have historically informed both penal/correctional practices and the treatment of the mentally ill; "rehabilitation;" "treatment;" "conditioning;" "freedom to —;" "freedom from —;" "privacy." The paramount question — Who controls/treats/conditions/demolishes Whom, Why, How, and Under What Considerations? — requires thoroughgoing analysis, not a mere observation that this question is troublesome.

Weppner's (1983) realistic, but pessimistic, conclusions regarding his participant-observer experiences at Matrix House needs to be studied assiduously by self-help programs because it replicates the sad happenings of Synanon:

> Therapeutic communities are not a radically new life-style. Utopian communities have existed in one form or another for hundreds of years and they have reached another period of fluorescence in the form of presentday ex-addict self-help groups. But, because of their inherent power, they also have the potential for immense corruption if not governed closely. Matrix House was not closely controlled and serves in its abject failure as testimony to the need for outside governance.

Dederich made himself the self-appointed monarch by fiat. He demanded conformity and compliance from everyone while he simultaneously liberated himself from any restriction and restraints. For awhile, Dederich functioned as an effective authoritarian leader. Hare (1962) offers some interesting insights regarding why it was possible for Dederich to be an effective leader:

> In industry or the army, however, where members anticipate forceful leadership from their superiors, a more authoritarian form of leadership results in a more effective group. . . [In these organizations] where members expect the leader to play an autocratic role, attemtps to introduce more democratic procedures usually result in member dissatisfaction and low productivity which is similar to that usually associated with autocratic leadership in a democratic culture.

A tragic double standard developed whereby Dederich and his coterie, who were able to amass absolute power, decided to apply different rules to themselves. It was not long before the decline started. Weppner (1973) describes the same phenomenon which destroyed Matrix House:

> The entrepreneurial directors were not subject to the same rules. They had discovered a new way to "jail." They had privileges that went beyond those of the ordinary inmate at Matrix. These privileges included unlimited freedom of movement, sex, superior quarters, travel as government employees, and unlimited authority over the lives of the members of the group. The effect on

the ordinary floor person cannot be empirically determined except to extrapolate from the splittee statistics. If a Matrix House member did not like the rules, he could leave.

Similarly, Dederich was able to free himself so that he could engage in any irresponsible and illicit behavior. Dederich arbitrarily and abruptly changed the rules of the game in a way in which Nietzsche would have approved. Nietzsche (1844-1900) anticipated a new generation of "supermen" who would be sufficiently powerful to free themselves from the petty and moral restraints which a weak and effete culture has created to stymie the strong. Nietzsche believed "superman" would rid the culture of the decadence and weakness. Superman would create a culture of strength and power which would rule those who would be unable to transcend their slave mentality. Dederich became vindictive and vituperative in an effort to discourage any overt or covert challenge to his assumed power by those he considered to be his moral inferiors. Some, who occupied top managerial positions and formed the inner sanctum of Synanon, agree that Dederich's downfall started when he refused to permit anyone either to confront him or to challenge his decision. It is possible, in retrospect, to document precisely when the empire of Synanon began to falter, i.e., when the founder became so consumed by power that he elevated himself to the Supreme ruler. Subtly, perhaps, almost imperceptively initially, Dederich decided he no longer needed to abide by the existing rules and regulations. Dederich issued the ultimatum that no one could confront him about anything he said or did. As soon as Dederich eliminated the checks and balances, his charisma was changed into grandiosity and finally disintegrated into delusional thinking when he believed he, in fact, had aspired to become the "Supreme Being" of Synanon who possessed the power to decide what was right and wrong for him empire.

Control is synonymous with power. Any external and intentional control or modification of individuals; thoughts, attitudes, and behavior is power. Any application of power or control, even in its most benevolent and benign form, can encroach upon the treasured concept of personal freedom which remains central to any democratic society. London (1969), who has discussed the ethics of behavior control, contends:

> The moral problem of behavior control is the problem of how to use power justly. . . The ethical challenge emphasized by behavior technology is that of how to perserve or enhance individual liberty under circumstances where its suppression will frequently be justified not only by the common welfare but also for the individual's happiness.

Even in its most idealistic form, any democracy requires leaders who retain some power to govern, i.e., to usurp some of the individual's fundamental freedom. The crucial concern is when leaders no longer use power as a potent instrument for helping individuals to help themselves but instead begin to violate the right (and trust) of others in their quest for personal power. The number of leaders who have been consumed and corrupted by the acquisition of power in the TC movement is far too great to be ignored. The Therapeutic Community needs to refine its accountability so that its leaders no longer can insulate themselves and delude others. Residents and staff must be encouraged to be aware of their respective power and obligation to provide realistic input so that leaders maintain their humility and humanity or else they will be corrupted by the very power which they created.

At the Second World Conference of Therapeutic Communities, Bassin (1978) warns: "An examination of the history of therapeutic communities reveals that . . . attacks of near psychotic behavior, insanity and craziness by staff has struck a high percentage . . . and the phenomenon deserves analysis and serious consideration for the development of remedial steps." The American self-help movement needs to consider the prophetic warning from Bassin, the ranking elder statesman, who had the expertise and vision to write the original proposal that resulted in the National Institute of Mental Health providing funds to create Daytop Lodge.

The only antidote to such power is a corresponding force which demands respect and equality. When no balance exists, the acquisition and justification of power can become a malignancy which is so all consuming that it destroys the democracy. Ideally, leaders will share power as soon as it is obvious individuals can govern themselves reasonably and responsibly. The Jones model can be implemented during the third phase of the self-help therapeutic community. When power is ethical and curative, it can be identified by the individual being encouraged to assume responsibility for his or her behavior. When leaders forget that, in the final analysis, in any democratic society the individual must retain the right for self-determination, they become tyrants and in so doing are enemies of the people.

CHAPTER 17

INTEGRATING MENTAL HEALTH PERSONNEL AND PRACTICES INTO A THERAPEUTIC COMMUNITY

JEROME F.X. CARROLL
BERNARD S. SOBEL

To CONSIDER the advantages and disadvantages of integrating mental health services into therapeutic community (TC) programs, it would seem helpful to first review some history. If the 1940s are used as a starting point, one would find that the MH field had relatively little interest and even less success in treating alcohol and/or drug dependent persons. The prevailing view of addiction held by most MH specialists at that time was tinged with moralistic overtones, as indicated by DSM I's classification of addiction as a form of sociopathic personality disorder.

During the 1950s and 1960s, the MH field made some adjustments in its thinking about addiction. The addicted patient was no longer automatically assigned a particular personality disorder, at least not that of "sociopath." On the other hand, a strong distinction was made between the alcohol and the drug dependent person — a reflection, perhaps, of society's greater tolerance for those disabled by their misuse of a legal substance (alcohol) versus those disabled by their misuse of illegal substances ("drugs"). For the most part, MH practitioners still were relatively ineffective in meeting the treatment needs of their addicted patients (Sobel, 1981).

The greatest treatment successes during this period were achieved through the self-help movement, principally Alcoholics Anonymous (AA). AA's officially stated attitude (AA, 1939)[1] toward the MH community was couched in positive terms; however, its operative attitude, at its best, was one of guarded, reluctant tolerance. At its worst, AA's attitude was one of outright intolerance and rejection of the relevance of MH services for those suffering from the disease of alcoholism.

The late 1960s and early 1970s saw an enormous growth in the self-help movement for addicted people, especially in the establishment of TCs for drug dependent persons. The MH field, for the most part, had relatively little to do with this development and watched with a mixture of relief (now there would be some place to which they could refer their addicted patients) and suspicion (word had filtered back about the "radical" forms of therapy used in the TCs).

Initial Impressions Gleaned From Early Contacts

When mental health practitioners[2] and TC staff[3] encountered one another, their early meetings were often marked by a guarded acceptance, mixed with suspicion and distrust. The TC staff tended to distrust the "theoretical orientation" of the MH practitioner. The TC staff were particularly offended by the MH belief that addiction was **simply** a symptomatic manifestation of a deeper underlying form of psychopathology.

The MH practitioners' emphasis on understanding the "whys" of behaviors (i.e., acquiring insight into the historical roots of contemporary destructive behavior patterns) was typically treated with disdain by many TC staff; TC staff would often refer to these insight-oriented therapies as "head games" and "mental masturbation." TC staff preferred to focus on the "here and now," in order to disrupt or eliminate overt destructive behavior patterns. They believed that the addicted person's underlying attitudes, values, and feelings would ultimately "catch up" to the induced, positive behavior changes.

The use of the diagnostic "labels" by MH practitioners was viewed as an impediment to treatment rather than an aid. TC staff were inclined to view these "labels" as stigmatizing people and/or creating artifical barriers between staff and residents of the TCs (Braginsky, 1975). Some diagnoses (e.g., "psychopath"), moreover, implied a very dismal prognosis which conflicted with the more positive attitude held by most TC staff regarding the possibility of recovery from an addiction (Carrol, 1975; 1978).

TC staff also believed that they "knew best" what was needed to help an addicted person to recover; "unless you've been there and worked through it, you really don't know what addiction is all about." There expertise had been acquired through "the school of hard knocks," and they were not about to take a subordinate position to anyone whose expertise rested solely on academic and professional training. Recovered staff bridled under the onus of having to continually struggle to gain full and equal status with non-recovered, professional staff members working in the same TC (DeBruce, 1975).

TCs which strove to operate on the principle of "participatory democracy" were also somewhat leery of taking in professional MH staff who were used to functioning in hierarchically structured systems in which they wielded maximal power and authority. The highly structured, relatively unchanging, discipline-specific job functions and responsibilities of the MH system also clashed with the more general, changing job functions and responsibilities which members of a TC typically undertook. For the most part, the former system produced specialists, the latter generalists.

From the MH practitioner's perspective, the TC staff's disdain for theory and "proven, traditional" therapeutic practices (e.g., individual, psychoanalytically oriented psychotherapy) was viewed as being reckless and/or almost totally without merit. The instantly claimed expertise of the recovered TC staff member was equally unacceptable to most MH practitioners.

The treatment modalities of the TC were also looked upon askance by many MH specialists. The use of confrontation techniques was often viewed by MH practitioners as being excessive, reeking of unresolved countertransference conflicts, and indiscriminately used, without due regard for a patient's readiness to profit from such an experience (Carroll, 1979). The lack of accountability and quality control also rankled the sensibilities of many MH health experts.

The second class status afforded non-recovered MH staff who did gain access to TCs was also unsettling. They were used to preferential treatment in systems designed to treat the emotionally distressed. To make matters worse, those relatively few MH specialists who were admitted, were often used as figureheads or "window dressing," as illustrated by programs which asked only that the MH health staff member "sign and sanction" what the "real" treatment staff had decided to do. Even when MH staff were given meaningful work to do with residents in TCs it was frequently only with the most severely disturbed, "at risk" residents.

The language and "street-smart" style of the TCs staff and residents was also difficult for many MH specialists to understand and adjust to; most MH staff were decidedly "non-street," traditional, middle class men and women. The distress and disdain for scholarship and credentials expressed by many in the TC also compounded the adjustment problems for most MH practitioners.

Finally, the explanations given by TC staff for the behavior of residents were often experienced by MH practitioners as being too simplistic and/or projections of the TC staff's own inner dynamics — a reflection of the assumption that "What worked for me, will surely work for them;" "This is what I felt and thought, it must be how they are feeling."

This is not to say that no positive impressions were gleaned from the mixing of MH specialists and TC staff. MH practitioners were favorably impressed by the high degree of personal commitment, zeal, and vitality which distinguished the TCs. The positive attitude which TC staff held for the possibility of recovery was also a welcomed change, especially for those MH practitioners who had worked with chronically disturbed mental patients in the backwards of overcrowded, under-funded MH facilities which, at best, often dispensed benevolent custodial care.

The comraderie of TC staff was also very impressive to most MH professionals. Genuine caring and liking seemed to be the norm for most TCs. Social support for staff was readily available, even for the staff member who could not verbalize the need for such support. This contrasted sharply with the role-dominated, highly-stylized, impersonal, "professional" interactions which occurred in most MH facilities.

The willingness of TC staff to experiment with new therapeutic procedures and techniques, to get personally involved in the delivery of services to residents (e.g., by sharing personal material, touching, confronting residents and risking being confronted in turn) was also exhilarating. Most MH specialists had been taught to maintain an aloof air of detachment/objectivity toward their patients, certainly not to get personally involved. They also typically worked in settings which offered limited opportunities to depart from traditional procedures, unless considerable bureaucratic and legal sanctions first were obtained.

The existence of a functioning, effective, truly interdisciplinary team, with no one discipline automatically exercising final authority, was also a welcome change for some MH professionals. In the TC, experience and competence — not title or degree — generally dictated who held the greatest authority within the team.

Finally, the TCs and their heterogeneous staff provided a living social laboratory where mental health people could encounter, study, and learn how to adapt to representatives from many diverse subcultures. The fact that residents exercised real power and control over their lives within the TCs, unlike most MH patients who were practically powerless, provided a unique and valuable learning environment which greatly benefited the MH staff, both professionally and personally.

Favorable impressions of MH specialists were also to be found among TC staff. MH staff were viewed as an additional, valued resource in coping with certain kinds of psychiatric crises (e.g., suicidal threats and attempts, psychotic breaks) and for their ability to identify, assess, and make helpful treatment recommendations for dealing with the brain damaged, retarded, or emotionally distressed resident.

Mental health specialists also brought with them useful therapeutic interventions not typically used in TCs (e.g., progressive relaxation, behavior modification, hypnotherapy, biofeedback, etc.). The MH specialist's ability to design and conduct research and evaluation on treatment outcome, therapeutic process, personality dynamics, and psychopathology were also appreciated, albeit usually after an initial period of considerable weariness.

The disciplined, cognitive approach taken by most MH specialists in most group problem-solving efforts also provided a welcomed counterpoint to the more affective, process-oriented, approach employed in most TCs. MH staff would sometimes provide a constructive break to prolonged, runaway destructive emotional diatribes which occasionally developed within the TC (e.g., in community meetings); for which most members of the community were grateful.

Finally, MH staff also provided TC staff with a viable, concrete example of positive, effective professionalism, which did much to counteract the prevailing TC view of MH professionals as cold, uncaring, ineffective, irrelevant entities. TC staff learned from their MH coworkers that it was possible to combine the need to maintain some emotional distince for the sake of being objective with the ability to personally engage residents to facilitate their rehabilitation. MH staff also encouraged and facilitated the efforts of TC staff to renew their education in pursuit of traditional degrees and credentials which have strengthened the TC movement.

Factors Favoring Greater Accommodations

Given the initial state of mutual distrust, misunderstanding and occasional outright hostility, albeit moderated by the less cogent, coexistent positive impressions, how could any constructive accommodation occur? There are several factors which predispose the MH and TC fields toward greater cooperation and reconciliation. One reason is reflected in the inextricable intermingling of addiction and MH problems to be found among nearly all substance abusers, typically distinguished by a self-concept laden with guilt and devoid of self-respect (Carroll, et al., 1978; 1982). With respect to specific psychiatric diagnoses, Sobel and Driscoll (1977), reported finding that 78 percent of the patient population at Eagleville Hospital (a facility which treats only substance abusers) had an associated psychiatric diagnosis: 72 percent of these diagnoses were personality disorders, 16 percent neurosis; 4 percent schizophrenia, and 3 percent affective disorders.

Carroll surveyed the medical records of one-half of the Eagleville Hospital population on a single day in October, 1983 (29 males; 28 females) and found that 76 percent of the males had a psychiatric diagnosis: 68 percent personality disorders; 23 percent personality disorders with a concommitant affective disorder, principally dysthymic disorder; and 9 percent affective disorders, again principally dysthymic. Among the women, 71 percent had a secondary psychiatric diagnosis; 35 percent personality disorders; 35 percent personality disorders with a concommitant affective disorder; 10 percent affective disorders; and 20 percent other. More serious diagnoses of psychopathology (e.g., borderline personality and schizoaffective disorder) were more frequently observed in the medical records of female patients than male patients.

De Leon (1976), Powell, et al., (1982) and Lewis, et al. (1983) similarly report a predominance of personality disorders and affective disorders among their diverse samples of substance abusers. In a study by Beck, et al. (1982) of male and female outpatient alcoholics, 45.7 percent of the patients reported that depression had preceded their alcoholic drinking; 39.1 percent stated that their alcoholism had preceded their experiencing depression; 15.2 percent denied ever being depressed. Kosten, et al., (1983) also reported finding a high incidence of depression among their sample of opiate-addicted patients.

A second factor likely to promote greater integration is that many of the most effective group and individual therapy strategems and techniques are commonly practiced by both MH and TC staff in their respective treatment centers. In addition, both MH and TC staff share a mutual desire to perfect their common therapeutic skills. These common practices and interests also serve as an important building block for further accommodation and cooperation.

The third reason favoring greater integration between the TC and MH fields relates to the political and economic realities of the 1980s. Today, more than ever before, there is greater demand for increased accountability and "proper" credentials, especially by insurance and government funding agencies supporting drug and/or alcohol programs. Thus, we see TC programs acquiring MH staff to enrich their staff development programs and to assist in the development and implementation of credentialing procedures for those TC staff without traditionally recognized credentials.

A fourth reason for greater accommodations is the growing realization that many people with serious emotional disorders **and** an addiction were "falling through the cracks," that is, no one wanted to treat them. MH facilities typically will not treat the addicted man or woman if the addiction is viewed as the primary problem; similarily, substance abuse programs are most reluctant to treat the "psychiatric patient." As more MH staff entered TCs, they developed tolerance and a more hopeful attitude in working with the addicted people. TC staff similarly learned that many "psychiatric" problems could be successfully managed and treated within the TC, which expanded their tolerance for such problems.

Finally, the increased contact between MH and TC staff and their successful teamwork in aiding countless addicted men and women to recovery has produced a growing mutual respect. This increased level of mutual respect undoubtedly has contributed to a more favorable attitude toward a greater degree of accommodation between MH and TC fields.

Potential Benefits to be Derived

Assuming a more positive and constructive accommodation is possible, what benefits are there to be realized by TCs? There are many. First, by adding MH specialists to the TC staff, either as permanent staff or part-time consultants, TCs will be able to address a broader range of treatment needs. Psychiatrists and psychologists, for example, have skills which would uncover issues which might otherwise go undetected in TCs without such services (e.g., subtle brain damage, varying degrees of retardation, dyslexia, incipient and/or residual psychotic processes, etc.). As a result of accomplishing a more thorough assessment of residents' assets and liabilities, more comprehensive and effective treatment plans can be developed and executed — to the benefit of the TC residents.

Another benefit is that many TC residents who experience periods of extreme emotional distress, with or without decompensation, could be retained in treatment, because the MH specialist, working closely and cooperatively with the TC staff, could devise treatment interventions to see them through their crisis situation. For example, by carefully and judiciously prescribing major antidepressants, antimania, or antipsychotic medications, a resident could soon be returned to the typical TC treatment regime and his/her medications either reduced gradually over time or discontinued all together. Without MH specialists, TC staff have no option but to transfer or discharge such residents from the TC.

A word of caution here, even with MH specialists on staff, TCs are limited with respect to the extent to which they can accommodate the seriously disturbed resident with psychiatric problems. Sobel and Antes (1975), in a study at Eagleville Hospital, reported finding that when the number of substance abusers with serious psychiatric complications exceeded 20 percent of the total resident population, the effectiveness of the treatment staff as a whole was adversely affected. The drain on staff and residents alike of expending the extra effort to accommodate the treatment needs of these residents was simply too great, even within a TC which had a psychology and a psychiatry department.

MH specialists can broaden the scope of services or therapeutic interventions which can be employed in the TC. Laying aside temporarily the debate about whether or not addicted people should ever take any medications (a rather extreme, absolutist argument taken by some within the substance abuse field), the authors believe there is a proper place for the judicious use of psychotropics and antagonists, such as antabuse and naltrexone, within the TC. In addition, the use of hypnotherapy, behavior modification, psychodrama, and other well established MH practices can only enhance the effectiveness of a TC's overall therapeutic program providing such diverse interventions are part of a well planned, executed and monitored program.

Another benefit of the merger of MH and TC personnel and practices is that TCs will be better able to evaluate the effectiveness of their treatment programs. Some MH specialists are very well trained in research and evaluation, and their skills would prove to be most helpful in attempting to objectively document the benefits derived from treatment (e.g., enhanced self-esteem, income earned and taxes paid, families re-united, etc.) versus common alternatives to treatment, such as being incarcerated or simply being free on the streets.

MH specialists can also enhance a TC's training and staff development program. Many MH staff have considerable teaching and training experience which can be readily utilized in an inhouse education/training program. Those TCs interested in promoting/encouraging staff to pursue traditional credentials will often discover that MH staff can, through their university affiliations, provide on-site college credit courses. Anyone who has observed the pride which a TC staff member takes in successfully completing such courses cannot help but be impressed with the results.

MH specialists can also help TCs to improve their quality control efforts, especially in reducing the incidents of misuse of therapeutic authority and prerogatives by staff. While granting the need for strong therapeutic interventions in treating addicted people (such as the use of confrontation), one must also acknowlege that the potential for abuse is always present in such strategies. Having MH staff assist in designing effective safeguards against the potential abuse of such practices cannot help but benefit TCs.

Finally, fewer addicted residents with serious emotional disorders (and psychiatric patients with a history of substance abuse) are failing to receive the treatment they need — whether residents in a TC or patients in a mental hospital. The increased contact between MH and TC practitioners has raised the consciousness level in both communities concerning this dual problem. Numerous modifications have been made in both programs to better accommodate the treatment needs of residents and patients with these problems. In addition, more and more programs are being designed specifically for this special population, with staff capable of coping with both the emotional and addiction problems.

Selected Illustrations of Positive Use for MH Practices Within the TC

Thirteen years ago, Dr. Carroll initiated a unique MH intervention at Eagleville Hospital referred to as "psychological feedback." This service entailed providing residents with complete, honest, and understandable "feedback" on the results of their psychological testing. The service was only given to those residents who requested it (about 85% of those tested and available to receive it). Residents were allowed to choose to receive their "feedback" in their therapy group (the over-whelmingly preferred location) or in an individual session with their psychologist. More than 10,000 Eagleville residents have requested and received "psychological feedback" during the time that this service was offered.

Reports received from residents and staff participating in psychological feedback sessions were most favorable. Residents reported the process helped them to better understand how certain repetitive behavior patterns kept them in their addiction. Group cohesion seemed to improve, since nearly everyone in the group could identify with some of the personality dynamics of the resident receiving feedback. Peers were better able to help the resident receiving feedback, because the process apparently helped them to obtain a clearer understanding of that resident.

Therapists appreciated the process, because they did not have to facilitate the feedback session, which constituted a welcomed "break." They also learned more about how personality dynamics contribute to addiction. The feedback process often succeeded in overcoming resident resistance and denial that had not yielded to the group therapy process.

Psychologists benefited in that the feedback process made their psychological testing more meaningful to the on-going therapeutic process. They felt more involved as a team member. Psychologists also learned to take greater care in formulating clinical impressions, since they had to explain and sometimes defend those impressions in the group therapy sessions.

Eagleville Hospital's modified TC[4] provided a variety of services through its Psychiatry Department (Sobel, 1976). Every resident was evaluated by a psychiatrist within 72 hours of his/her admission. Whenever significant psychopathology was identified, residents were placed on alert/observation (A/O) status[5] (Sobel & Antes, 1975). A/O residents received closer supervision and support[6] until their condition improved, at which time they were removed from A/O status and entered fully into the mainstream of daily activities within the community.

Psychiatrists also provided individual psychotherapy to residents undergoing an emotional crisis. These sessions were typically of limited duration and supplemented rather than superseded the group therapy process. If the resident required long-term individual psychotherapy, the psychiatrist would arrange to have the resident transferred to a psychiatric facility until the resident's condition improved and he/she could return to the community.

Psychiatrists routinely consulted with staff regarding a variety of therapeutic management decisions. Psychiatrists were particularly help-ful in helping staff assess a resident's "acting out" potential for suicide and/or assault, as well as differentiating between "lazy apathy" and the type of lethargy and inertia seen in severe depressive states. These dif-ferentials were viewed as helpful to the Eagleville staff in deciding when to intensify the confrontation of manipulative residential behavior without medications, and when to "back off" confrontation in favor of "nursing and nurturing," without medications, to promote further ego decompensation.

A special case can be made for the psychiatrist's role in making dif-ferential diagnoses pertaining to the management of borderline states. The transitory dissociative-psychotic reaction experienced by the alco-holic is commonly referred to as the "dry-drunk." The patient expe-riences vague paranoid ideations, sleep disturbances, fleeting bedtime hallucinatory episodes, and free-floating anxiety. This usually occurs af-ter three to four weeks of abstinence. Others report this phenomenon af-ter many months of sobriety.

For many, these symptoms of distress come about as a result of inten-sive introspection, temporary ego regression, and the uncovering and working through of significant areas of conflict. For others, this symp-tom picture represents early psychotic disorganization of an underlying schizophrenic process, formerly self-medicated with alcohol and/or other drugs. The phenomenon cannot be taken lightly or attributed to an extended "hang-over." Psychiatric consultation is most useful in de-ciding the best course of treatment for residents presenting with these symptoms.

A borderline state similar to the "dry drunk" occurs in some recov-ering drug dependent residents. The characteristic symptoms are attrib-uted to the active addictive use of amphetamines or hallucinogens. The symptoms include: pressure of speech, blocking of thoughts, paranoid ideation, and disorientation as to time and place. One may also see states of manic-type behavior, lability of affect with temporary elation and euphoria. This borderline state is sometimes mistakenly interpreted as a positive therapeutic "break-through," (i.e., the crumbling of un-wanted defenses). Again, careful consideration must be given to the pro-dromal signs and symptoms of psychotic decompensation which usually necessitates scheduling a psychiatric consultation.

Eagleville psychiatrists were also responsible for prescribing and monitoring all psychotropic medications. The majority of residents re-ceiving such medications presented with intensive borderline states of anxiety, depression, and dysphoria. The degree of disorganization, loss of ego defenses, and poor reality testing indicated an imminent danger of a psychotic states. Less intense states of anxiety and depression with more intact ego mechanism were treated with psychotherapy and modifications in group interaction.

At Eagleville, the use of low to moderate doses of phenothiazines, (e.g., thioridazine, Mellaril, up to approximately 125 mg./24 hours) or other antipsychotic medications (e.g., haldoperidol, Haldol up to approximately 15 mg./24 hours) proved to be very effective in treating these borderline psychotic crises. Most other non-psychotic psychotropic medications (barbiturates, narcoleptics, benzodiazepines) are prone to "abuse," therefore they were seldom prescribed. One must also remember that use of antianxiety agents does not protect against psychotic decompensation.

Since a major therapeutic concern reflects the resident's ability to function optimally during the waking hours, states of medicated drowsiness or somnolence were ill-tolerated, especially by the non-medical, treatment staff. This type of dozing was interpreted as the equivalent of addictive behavior of "nodding-out." To minimize this phenomenon, approximately one-half to three-fourths of each calculated 24-hour dose was given at bedtime, minimizing or negating the need for "sleep medications," since a significant number of patients also have sleep disturbances.

Medications also played a significant role at Eagleville Hospital in preventing seizures which have the potential to be life threatening. Fortunately, most seizures occur during the detoxification phase of treatment. To guard against such seizures, residents with documented histories of seizure were prescribed medication, such as Dilantin with phenobarbital. Typically such medication was given for a specified period of time with dosage decreased over time.

Residents diagnosed as having status epilepticus, a condition in which one seizure compounds on another, leading in some instances to fatal heart attacks or cardiac irregularities, were prescribed intravenous Valium.

In all cases involving the use of medication, the key to success in guarding against addictive manipulations for medications lies in promoting a constructive, ongoing, rational dialogue between the non-medical and medical staff who **both** must carefully monitor the behavior of the resident receiving such treatment. When this is successfully accomplished, the proper use of medications should present no challenge to a TC's commitment to an abstinence ethic.

Potential Liabilities of Integration

The pressure to create "medically oriented" treatment programs, while enhancing a program's potential for funding/reimbursement for services, could well undermine the egalitarian, participatory-democracy style that characterizes most TCs. In its place, a medically-dominated, rigidly structured decision-making process could well emerge. (Others would counter that the decision-making processes of a TC wastes considerable time, gives equal voice to the ill-informed as to the well-informed, and generally is not very efficient).

A related variation on this theme is the breakdown of a true interdisciplinary term effort which often accompanies the institution of a medically dominated program. Since the physician has "the final say," members of the team eventually feel less and less responsible for and valued in contribution to "team decisions," leading some members to withdraw from the process, while others express their frustration and anger through passive-aggressive acts of sabotage.

Along with a greater integration of MH staff into the TC will often come a usually tacit commitment to the disease-oriented medical model. This model, in its extreme application, tends to "blame the victim" (Ryan, 1971) while typically ignoring environmental problems and stressors which play a significant role in most addicted people's "problems-in-living." The etiology is assumed to lie almost exclusively within the resident's disturbed intrapsychic processes of conflict and frustration. In addition, many adhering to this point of view would argue that only the highly trained mental health professional is best qualified to treat such problems (Carroll, 1975).

MH specialists are especially enamored with the art of diagnosis, yet too often diagnoses have proven to be more of a hindrance than aid to the recovery process. Unfortunately, diagnostic labels may be interpreted by some residents and staff to be a final negative authoritative judgment which induces a self-fulfilling prophecy of failure and hopelessness. When such diagnoses are provided by staff who are precevied to be "the modern high priests of mental health," (Braginsky & Braginsky, 1973), some staff will be much disinclined to question or challenge the validity and authenticity of the diagnosis.

Diagnoses have also been criticized for implying a greater level of knowledge about a person's disorder than is actually the case. Having said all of this, the authors wish to point out that making a diagnosis will not automatically result in injury to an individual, only that without proper precautions, the potential for harm is always present.

Many staff in TCs share the popularly held belief that the medical and MH fields are guilty of over-prescribing psychotropic medications, and indeed, there is evidence that supports that perception (Bowes, 1974; Hasday & Karch, 1981; Rudestam & Tarbell, 1981). Studies such as Rosser's (1982), however, suggest that the problem may be somewhat overstated.

To complicate matters, many staff in TCs (especially staff who have achieved sobriety through an abstinence oriented program) believe that addicted people in treatment should take no substances, including medications prescribed by physicians. Physicians and psychiatrists typically have worked in MH facilities where the use of psychotropic medications is considered normal and proper and are not inclined to doubt the appropriateness or efficacy of such treatment. Even in cases where the prescription is accomplished in a judicous and sensitive manner, conflict can occur.

MH specialists also are inclined to emphasize the historical roots of maladaptive behaviors, including addiction. Thus, they tend to search out the presumed underlying causes of addiction believing that "insight" will lead to positive behavioral changes. TC staff focus more on the present and stress eliminating addictive behaviors and developing behaviors conducive to sobriety. This clash of time perspectives and emphasis too can create conflict within the TC.

Methods of management and decision-making are often at variance between MH practitioners and TC staff which all too often creates considerable opportunities for misunderstanding and exasperation. Many TC staff extend their own therapeutic experience into their management style. For these staff members, full expression of one's feelings must occur before any rational weighing of alternatives and final decision is reached. The venting of affect and processing of how decisions were made are perceived as one of the principal means by which a cohesive and egalitarian TC is held together.

MH staff typically bring a more structured decision-making process into the TC. Many MH staff tend to view the full expression of emotions as a "therapeutic technique" rather than a problem-solving or decision-making modality. Also, many MH staff used to functioning at higher decision-making levels may see this egalitarian approach as an excessively inefficient method of management.

MH specialists with advanced degrees and credentials, MDs, DOs, PH.Ds, MSWs, etc., can generally command higher salaries than staff working in TCs with less education and/or no credentials or credentials with lower market values. This inevitably creates conflicts and resentments. No matter how strong the commitment to egalitarianism, the reality of the employment market place will prevail.

The conflict can be especially strong when lower paid staff perceive themselves as doing more vital work within the TC (e.g., running extended therapy sessions and marathon groups) than higher paid staff (e.g., psychiatrists doing mental status exams or psychologists doing psychological testing).

To a certain extent, economic and political forces have combined to require TCs to be more accountable to external regulatory and funding sources. This typically necessitated adding "properly educated and credentialled mental health specialists" to the staff. To the extent that the existing staff understands and accepts the inevitability of this development, the conflicts and resentments will at least be minimized.

Suggestions for Maximizing Potential Benefits

Considerable problems can be avoided if TCs desirous of adding MH specialists to their staff recruit professionals who already have considerable experience working with addicted people, and even more desirable, knowledge and experience with TCs. Given that the pool of available MH specialists with such backgrounds is somewhat limited, then TCs should take the time and make a concerted effort to design a comprehensive orientation program for MH professionals who are invited to join the community. Time and care spent in properly educating and orienting such staff will pay big dividends down the line.

While acknowledging the fact that orientation and indoctrination are essential for all newly acquired staff to facilitate their entry into and acceptance by the TC, special recognition must be afforded to some of the delicate system's dynamics triggered by the arrival of a new MH specialist. Veteran TC staff are typically asked to bear the brunt of this orientation and training of new arrivals, in addition to carrying out their many other duties. This can lead to their feeling used and/or abused; after all these MH specialists are already supposed to be "professionally trained." This potential problem can be ameliorated in several ways: 1) reduce the trainers' normal workload; 2) provide some salary increment to the trainers; and 3) require the MH specialist to reciprocate with some training in his/her area of expertise to the existing staff.

The reciprocation of training suggested above may also promote the understanding and acceptance of the specialized services introduced into the TC by the MH professional. Where these new services yield success, these results should be brought to the attention of the entire community. Once staff see the value of the new MH interventions, there usually is a desire for more of these services.

As the MH professionals become familiar with the positive utilization of the non-traditional interventions typically employed in the TC, they too will be positively motivated to integrate these techniques into their own practices. The demonstration of successful interventions, then, is the binding force which ultimately brings new and veteran staff members together.

A word of caution regarding the selection and utilization of staff. Responsible staff selection and utilization is the key ingredient for any program — especially the TC whose principal strength rests on the strength and character of its staff, regardless of their position, authority, and responsibility. Just as credentials alone do not guarantee that a MH specialist will function effectively within a TC (or any human services setting), the same holds true for the recovered TC staff. Recovery from one's own addiction through a personal therapeutic experience does not automatically qualify a person to become an effective deliverer of services and/or manager within the TC. Each program must set its own high standards for staff recruitment, selection, and training for all positions. To accomplish this objective, programs must be wary of making prejudicial assumptions of competence or incompetence about any category of individuals who would be considered for hire.

Another programmatic device for insuring a successful merger of MH and TC personnel and procedures is to create a strong internal staff development program. Staff lacking in formal education and/or without professional degrees and credentials should be the principal beneficiaries of these programs. Anyone who has witnessed the positive personal and professional growth realized through such programs knows of what we write. The authors believe the earning of "proper" credentials and degrees is the only legitimate equalizer which will overcome the salary discrepancy problem previously cited, as well as ameliorate much of the suspicion and wariness that exists between MH and TC staff members.

Blending the Best of the Two Camps

The most important factor in maximizing benefits and minimizing liabilities is for the top managers to be fully cognizant of the need to blend the best of the MH and TC approaches to treatment of the addicted person. To accomplish this task, top management must be intimately familiar with the strengths and weaknesses of the two systems. Since no one individual is likely to possess such knowledge, it follows that a planning committee, balanced in terms of numbers and power, representing both the MH and TC points of view, should seek to accomplish the ideal blend of the two perspectives and procedures.

TCs have been particularly effective in teaching addicted men and women "responsible concern" through their use of a participatory democracy style in their decision-making processes and through the use of behavioral contracts and feedback. This element should be retained. Their use of strong, confrontational therapeutic interventions which were designed to penetrate highly resistive defenses and images should also be preserved. The emphasis placed on uncovering and working through deep-seated emotional traumas and conflicts should also be retained. Their insistence on not neglecting the emotional element of the decision-making process also has merit. Finally the employment of recovered staff as living models of hope and successful struggle against the ravages of addiction is a must for retention.

The key to retaining the most salient and effective elements of the TC approach lies in developing an effective quality assurance monitoring system. Here the MH specialist can be especially helpful in designing and implementing such a system. Many of the mistakes made by TCs in the past can be traced to the lack of an internal, objective, quality assurance monitoring system. Such systems offer the potential of preventing excesses and insuring a continuing refinement in program policies and procedures.

What is at stake at this vital historical juncture is the very survival of the TC's unique form of treatment which has demonstrated an unquestioned ability to successfully rehabilitate the chemically addicted person — a disabled individual whom many experts, both within and without the MH field once had abandoned as hopelessly incurable. The challenge to us all is to help preserve and improve upon the TC movement during this difficult period of economic and political adversity. To this end, this chapter was written and dedicated.

Notes

1. "But this does not mean that we disregard human health measures. God has abundantly supplied this world with fine doctors, psychologists, and practitioners of various kinds. Do not hesitate to take your health problems to such persons. Most of them give freely of themselves, that their fellows may enjoy sound minds and bodies. Try to remember that though God has wrought miracles among us, we should never belittle a good doctor or psychiatrist. Their services are often indispensable in treating a newcomer and following his case afterward (p. 147)."
2. MH practitioners typically were non-recovered, held advanced degrees (e.g., MDs, DOs, PH.Ds, MAs, etc.,), had little experience working with addicted patients, and rarely had had any previous contact with TCs.
3. TC staff typically were recovered, seldom had advanced degrees (some had not finished high school), and tended to use their own treatment experience and recovery as the "life experience credentialing" necessary to treat others.
4. In 1983, Eagleville Hospital began to deemphasize the therapeutic community nature of its program in favor of a more traditional medical-psychiatric model of treatment.
5. Residents were placed on A/O status for extreme anxiety, depression, suicidal ideation, paranoia, dissociative reactions, potential for violence, and sudden and severe mood change.
6. This support often included a "group watch" which entailed having two members of the resident's group present at all times. The group watch typically lasted for one or two days. Residents participating in the group watch typically reported experiencing a sense of accomplishment and greater group cohesion.

CHAPTER 18

THERAPEUTIC COMMUNITIES WITHIN PRISONS

HARRY K. WEXLER

INTRODUCTION

THE THERAPEUTIC community (TC) approach has significant value for prison rehabilitation efforts. Some central reasons that TCs are effective for prison inmates and can function in prison environments are outlined below.

Prisons are usually highly conservative institutions, primarily concerned with order and control and opposed to anything that disturbs the status quo. The general authoritarian orientation of TCs is not at variance with the conservative prison outlook. The TC's strong emphasis on following rules, clearly delineated roles and responsibilities as well as a hierarchical authority structure is not contrary to general prison life.

Although inmates usually volunteer for TC programs there remains a basic contradiction between the general involuntary inmate status and the need to establish therapeutic conditions (e.g., trust, honesty, openness, etc.) for positive growth. The prison TC facilitates the development of a therapeutic environment by utilizing counselors with drug and criminal histories as primary role models and change agents. These parprofessional counselors are often successful graduates of TCs and display a degree of inspiration since they have experienced the benefits of the treatment. A certain amount of inspired dedication is necessary to motivate apathetic inmates and is highly preferable to the more typical bureaucratic attitudes (e.g., boredom, ineptitude and helplessness) found in traditional correctional counseling units.

Therapeutic communities do not simply deliver services. Rather, they elicit inmate involvement in several important ways. Since participants usually live together in a segregated unit there are many experiences of sharing and working out problems that lead to the development of meaningful relationships. Since values of honesty, responsibility, caring and helpfulness are integral to the TC experience inmates begin to internalize these values over the course of treatment. Changes in value structures are essential to meaningful and lasting rehabilitation.

Prisons are depressing environments and the inmates' culture engenders survival concerns, pessimism and cynical attitudes. In contrast, the TC communicates a sense of optimism; for example, if participants work hard and develop competencies there are few limits to ambition. There is a strong implicit (staff role models) and an explicit message that it is possible to rise out of the mire of social deprivation, prejudice and personal inadequacies. Participants are trained to tolerate frustration and develop persistent work habits which are necessary for positive achievements.

BACKGROUND LITERATURE

The most extensive review of the outcomes of various prison-based rehabilitative efforts for criminal offenders was produced by Lipton, Martinson and Wilks (1975). The overall conclusion was that ". . . the field of corrections has not as yet found satisfactory ways to reduce recidivism by significant amounts" (p. 627). Other reviews (e.g., Bailey, 1966; Adams, 1975) do not contradict this pessimistic conclusion.

Reasons for the lack of documented notable effectiveness of correctional treatment include: a limited number of relevant studies which are of generally poor quality; the present narrow range of treatment techniques; the fundamental incompatability of punitive correctional environments and rehabilitation programs seeking to facilitate positive client change; and a lack of connection between both treatment and evaluation with theory (Lipton, et al., 1975).

A theoretical rationale for the establishment of TCs within prison is derived from outcome research on community-based TCs. An important finding is that successful outcomes (reduced crime and substance abuse and increased employment) are related to the time spent in treatment (De Leon, 1984; De Leon et al., 1979; Simpson, 1979, 1980). In fact, residents who were sent to the program by the courts had a better success rate then volunteers. However, community TCs produce excessively high dropout rates which limit their effectiveness to the relatively few clients who remain at least six months in the program (De Leon, 1979). One of the justifications for the establishment of the "Stay 'N Out" program was to test the efficacy of the time-in-program variable within an environment where residents are likely to stay at least six months. It was expected that inmates would find the program unit considerably more desirable than regular prison units.

Although a number of TCs within prison settings have been established in state and federal prisons (NIDA, 1981) there has been almost no outcome research conducted. A study conducted by Lynn and Nash (1975) assessed changes in arrest rates for a total of 173 inmates who attended seven prison-based programs. Four of these programs were TCs based on the traditional Synanon model, two were counseling programs and one was a drug-free residential program. The study did not find significant differences in arrest rates between any of the programs and a comparison group. However, a more extensive analysis of the data (Des Jarlais and Wexler, 1979) found that two of the four TCs did significantly better than the comparison group. Within the community, TCs have been shown to be effective with clients who have extensive criminal histories (De Leon et al., 1972, 1979; De Leon et al, 1981; Nash, 1973, 1976; System Science, 1973; Sells et al., 1976; Wilson and Mandelbrot, 1977).

The remainder of this chapter will focus on the "Stay 'N Out" TC which is a model of a successful prison-based rehabilitation program. A program description will be followed by a summary of evaluation research conducted a "Stay 'N Out" and a discussion of how the program has developed important conditions necessary for effective rehabilitation within the prisons.

"STAY 'N OUT" PROGRAM DESCRIPTION

The "Stay 'N Out" program was founded in 1977 as a joint venture between New York Therapeutic Communities, New York Department of Correctional Services, New York Division of Substancs Abuse Services, and the New York Division of Parole in 1977. The successful cooperation between these agencies is a primary reason for the success and longevity of the program. A male program (capacity of 62) is located at the Arthur Kill Correctional Facility on Staten Island and the female program (capacity of 31) is housed at Manhattan based Bayview Correctional Facility.

Inmates selected for the programs are recruited at State correctional facilities. The criteria for selection are: history of drug abuse, at least 18 years of age, evidence of positive institutional participation, and no history of sex crimes or mental illness.

The programs at Arthur Kill and Bayview are TCs modified to fit into a correctional institution. "Stay 'N Out" clients are housed in units segregated from the general prison population. They eat in a common dining room, however, and attend morning activities with other prisoners. The length of treatment is from six to nine months. Most program staff are graduates of community-based TCs as well as ex-offenders with prison experience who act as "role models" demonstrating successful rehabilitation. The course of treatment is viewed as a developmental growth process with the inmate becoming an increasingly responsible member of society.

During the first phase of treatment, the major clinical thrust involves observation and assessment of client needs and problem areas, and re-education and orientation of the client to the lifestyle of the therapeutic community. Re-education and orientation occurs through individual counseling, encounter sessions and seminars.

During the second phase of treatment, participants are placed in positions of increasing responsibility. Encounter groups and counseling sessions are more indepth and focus on the areas of self-discipline, self-worth, self-awareness, respect for authority, and acceptance of guidance for problem areas. Seminars take a more intellectual nature. Debate is encouraged to enhance self-expression and to increase self-confidence.

The re-entry process includes close cooperation with the Department of Social Services, Office of Vocational Rehabilitation, and private agencies. This is intended as a bridge for the residents in achieving economic, personal and social adjustment. Upon release, participants are encouraged to seek further substance abuse treatment at cooperating community-based TCs.

"STAY 'N OUT" EVALUATION FINDINGS

Since the inception of "Stay 'N Out," the New York State Division of Substance Abuse Services Bureau of Cost Effectiveness and Research has been monitoring the programs and conducting evaluation studies which are summarized by Wexler and Chin (1981). Data is collected on basic client flow, client background characteristics, types of termination, psychological testing, environmental assessment and outcome. Selected results of these efforts are summarized below.

An extensive battery of psychological tests has been utilized to assess client changes in treatment. These include the MMPI and the Tennessee Self-Concept Scale. Clients were tested within one month of admission and again approximately six months later. Overall, the psychological results indicated a variety of improvements in psychological functioning for males and females who experienced approximately six months of therapeutic community treatment while in prison. Earlier research (De Leon, 1984) in community-based TCs has shown that positive changes on psychological measures are related to successful client outcomes. For example, improvements in self-concept and decreases in depression were related to decreases in crime drug use as well as improved employment status.

A standardized instrument which assesses staff and client program environmental perceptions (Moos, 1974) is administered twice a year to monitor the quality of the treatment environment and provide feedback to staff and clients. Previous studies have shown that positive perceptions of program environments are related to positive client outcomes.

Overall, the treatment environments of both programs are perceived as highly positive and treatment oriented. The test scores were significantly more positive than results reported for typical prison units and resemble TC data reported in the literature (Wexler and Lostlen, 1979). These data demonstrate that TC environments have been successfully implemented and maintained with the Authur Kill and Bayview prisons.

One of the "Stay 'N Out" program goals is to encourage clients to continue treatment in community-based TCs after release. A study of 109 positive male program completions showed that 59 entered community TCs. The six-month drop out rate for these clients was 49 percent which was considerably lower than 72 percent six-month average drop out rate for all TCs within New York State (New York State Division For Substance Abuse Services, 1980).

Parole outcome data were obtained for all clients who terminated from the Arthur Kill (N = 110) and Bayview (N = 43) programs prior to 12/31/79 and have been placed on parole status. Data were also obtained for two comparison groups, consisting of individuals who had been on the Arthur Kill (N = 115) and Bayview (N = 16) waiting list but were never admitted to the programs. Comparisons were made between program and comparison groups to ascertain their degree of similarity. There were no significant differences found between program and comparison groups for "time at risk" (average range from 18 to 21 months), age, ethnicity, religion, education, marital status, occupational level, narcotic and alcohol abuse history, number of prior arrests and convictions, and severity of crime leading to current incarceration.

The parole revocation rate for the Arthur Kill program males was 6 percent which was significantly lower than the 19 percent found for the male comparison group. In addition, none of the Bayview program females had their parole status revoked, as compared with 6 percent of the comparison females. These data indicate that participation in the "Stay 'N Out" program leads to a reduction in the incidence of parole revocation. These preliminary findings, however, need to be replicated with larger samples over longer periods at risk.

CONDITIONS FOR SUCCESSFUL REHABILITATION

The "Stay 'N Out" prison TC meets five important conditions for a successful rehabilitation outlined by Dr. Douglas S. Lipton (whose 1977 comprehensive review of the literature is often cited in defense of the "rehabilitation is impossible within prisons" position) at the 1983 Bellevue Forensic Psychiatry Conference. The conditions include: an isolated treatment unit; motivated participants; a committed and competent staff; adequate treatment duration; and, continuity of care that extends into the community. Discussion of how these conditions were met by the program should be useful in developing effective rehabilitation programs within other correctional settings. In addition, several important program developments will be discussed which help illuminate the difficulties of instituting and maintaining effective rehabilitation programming within prisons.

One of the major reasons "Stay 'N Out" has been able to provide conditions for an effective program is it's independence. The program is an autonomous organization which has been successful in gaining cooperation and support from other important agencies (e.g., New York State Division of Parole, New York State Department of Correctional Services, New York Division of Substance Abuse Services, many large therapeutic communities and the national organization of Therapeutic Communities of America).

Independence has allowed the program to enhance its negotiating position with other agencies through the formation of alliances. For example, although funding is exclusively provided through a contract with corrections, the considerable support received from other agencies improves the bargaining position of "Stay 'N Out." Conversely, support received from corrections helps the program negotiate issues, with other agencies.

Independence also enhances program credibility with inmates. Since a basic therapeutic task is to gain credibility and trust it is mandatory that counselors are not perceived as employees of corrections. In fact, inmates and program staff show the common concern of maximizing their independence from the values and coercive authority found among the general population. Pride is taken in program membership.

Isolated Unit

"Stay 'N Out" is located on isolated units within the prison. The program is a show place for the prison administration. Most important visitors to the prison are taken on tours of the units. Upon entering one of the units visitors are immediately impressed with how neat and clean it appears. Each bedroom is attractively decorated and looks well cared for. All program participants are clean and well mannered. They are very willing to discuss their personal lives and/or program. Their perceptions of the program are consistently positive although they don't hesitate to mention deficiencies.

An issue of trust was provoked by the placement of a program, administered by an outside group, onto an isolated unit within the prison. Inmates and correctional personnel were suspicious and disturbed by the intrusion of a positive program which created a bright and attractive environment that was a glaring contrast to the surrounding poor prison conditions.

The mistrust of prison inmates and staff was handled in several ways. Close working relationships were developed with the prison administration. Several higher echelon administrators who were honestly interested in rehabilitation were invited to identify with the program accomplishments. These administrators were proud to show visitors and their correctional superiors the good programming taking place under their auspices and guidance.

The support of correctional officers was earned by involving officers assigned to the units. These unit officers were deeply impressed by the dedication of program staff, clarity of program values and positive observed changes among participating inmates. Over time, officers who were exposed to the program communicated their positive impressions to the rest of the prison staff. In addition, the program fielded sports teams, sponsored events (e.g., Christmas parties) and encouraged it's inmate members to participate in other positive prison programs (e.g., college courses).

Gaining the trust of general population inmates within the host prison and other prisons was necessary to provide a pool of future recruits. That the program was very successful in winning inmate confidence was confirmed by a continous long waiting list. Inmates have a well established informal communication network ("grape vine") that extends throughout the entire New York State correctional system. The specific ways that the program gained a positive statewide reputation among inmates is described in the recruitment section below.

Motivated Participants

The primary reason "Stay 'N Out" was highly popular among inmates was that it demonstrated an ability to deliver on it's promises. Inmates, who are generally quite cautious and cynical, scrutinize a program very carefully before committing themselves. The program has been able to keep the most important promise which is favorable review by the Parole Board for it's members. Through continuous efforts "Stay 'N Out" has maintained a high degree of positive visibility among the Board members. These efforts have included presentations to the Board, cooperative relations with Institutional and Field Parole Officers and good communication with the Executive Officer of Parole.

The promise that "Stay 'N Out" is capable of successfully rehabilitating inmates has also been publicized. Research that has demonstrated successful outcome has been actively disseminated. Several successful graduates have returned to the program as paid staff and other successful clients have returned to visit.

Since motivation is very low or entirely absent among prison inmates, it is not a requirement for admission. However, the program considers the inspiration and maintenance of motivation for success a primary objective. Explication of how motivation is encouraged is offered in the following sections which discuss program staff and the need for a six month minimum of immersion in a treatment process.

Committed and Competent Staff

Ex-addicts and ex-offenders who have successfully completed TC treatment comprise most of the program staff.

An essential requirement for an effective treatment staff is the personal strength and integrity gained from completing treatment and succeeding. Counselors who meet this requirement are inspired and deeply believe in the treatment process and their own power to facilitate and guide positive development.

Staff members who are willing to work for relatively low pay and remain committed to the program for significant durations are usually people who are still actively involved in the rehabilitation process. They have recently completed treatment and need to consolidate their gains and altered identities by helping others achieve similar growth. Often, these counselors lack the skills and experience to demand greater pay in other forms of employment. Although these staff members are talented and highly committed, care must be taken not to continue employing them when they outgrow the job. If ex-addict/offenders stay too long it usually reinforces negative dependencies which hinders their effectiveness.

The fact that staff members come from similar backgrounds to the inmates enables them to serve as credible role models. The successful rehabilitation demonstrated by counselors is a strong impetus to client motivation. The staff provides undeniable proof that the treatment can work if one fully participates in the process.

Adequate Treatment Duration

Program staff strongly believe that a minimum of six months of treatment is necessary for the establishment of significant client changes. Adequate time is needed in the various program structures (e.g., encounter groups, seminars, job assignments, etc.) to break down negative self concepts (e.g., tough guy) and facilitates the development of social maturity. Clients are continually involved in program-induced cycles of stress and adaptation (new learning) designed to foster increasing levels of competency. Over time participants hopefully internalize values of honesty, integrity, responsibility and concern for others. The course of treatment is designed sequentially so that clients earn reinforcements (privileges and status) for demonstrating increasingly mature behavior. Client success and subsequent reinforcements serve to promote and maintain motivation.

A central therapeutic component is the formation of a positive network of staff and peers that forms the bridge into the community. It is truism in penology that inmates who return to the old environment are likely to also return to prison. The formation of a new network that extends from the prison program to the community helps decrease recidivism. Description of the program aftercare network is presented below.

Continuity of Care

Programs that simply refer ex-inmates to community service programs such as job training have very little success because they ignore several critical realities. Criminal justice clients generally suffer from overwhelming social defenses and need to undergo a great deal of training and development to become socially adequate and earn a decent living. The problem is that very high levels of fear and anxiety are elicited by the difficult tasks facing ex-inmates and most individuals strenuously avoid situations that engender such feelings of weakness. A great deal of personal integrity and support is needed for these clients to achieve successful integration into the community.

"Stay 'N Out" has developed a network of cooperative community TCs that recruit their clients. Community TC staff regularly visit the program and develop personal relationships with clients. Community programs that are most successful with "Stay 'N Out" clients have modified their procedures to meet the special needs of ex-inmates. Clients who complete "Stay 'N Out" and enter the community TC network are provided with the integrity support system needed to enable successful passage into the community.

CONCLUSIONS

The effectiveness of TC treatment within prison, as exemplified by the "Stay 'N Out" program, directly challenges the wide-spread belief that it is impossible to implement effective prison-based rehabilitation programs. It is hoped that the discussion of how the "Stay 'N Out" program developed will suggest strategies for the development of other effective prison TCs. Some of the conditions that increase the likelihood of success include: isolation of the treatment unit; inspiration and maintenance of inmate motivation; staff who are committed and competent; adequate treatment duration; and, continuity of care that helps the client re-enter the community.

The TC model holds great promise for effective rehabilitation of felons. The approach is one of self-help that employs credible role models (ex-addicts and ex-offenders) who have successfully helped themselves. The national network of TCs within the field of substance abuse comprises a competent staff who are experienced with criminal justice clients. The TC provides a well defined, structured program that engages participants in pro-social behaviors and strongly discourages negative values and conduct. The hierarchical authoritarian TC approach is uniquely compatible with correctional environments. Careful attention to the special needs of inmates and creative approaches to the inherent difficulties of prison rehabilitation will result in more extensive utilization of prison-based TCs.

CHAPTER 19

THE THERAPEUTIC COMMUNITY: A PLAN FOR CONTINUED INTERNATIONAL DEVELOPMENT

JAMES T. ZIEGENFUSS, JR.*

THE CONCEPT of therapeutic community appeared in the professional literature some thirty years ago. Beginning in England at the onset of World War II, the notion of a model of psychosocial treatment in a group and community framework is now expanding and gaining acceptance by both the professional and the greater communities.

Initiated in a traditional medical unit designed to treat cardiac neurosis, the sociological and psychological emphasis in the unit soon led to a redesign of the social organization and the use of group and community treatment. Although that first unit was replaced by one designed for returning British prisoners of war in 1945, it began the evolution of therapeutic community attitudes, values, and beliefs. Maxwell Jones assumed the leadership role in both the actual practice and the recording of the experiences (Jones, 1952) and continues that role today in the mental health field (see Jones 1979).

Simultaneously, another British group was moving toward the therapeutic community concept. The use of group psychology and group dependency was further discussed by Menninger (1946), Main (1946) and Bridger (1946) in what were two of the earliest reports on the therapeutic community known as the Northfield Experiment. It is enough to note here that the therapeutic community (hereafter TC) concept first ap-

*James T. Ziegenfuss, Jr., as the author, would like to thank Drs. Maxwell Jones, Alan Kraft, and Stuart Whiteley for their helpful reviews. Preparation of this paper was supported in part by the TRW and AMP Corporations in Harrisburg, PA.

peared in two British settings as a response to psychoneuroses. Its general history has been thoroughly recounted by Manning (1975, 1976). Concept development also occurred in still a third stream. The history of addictions treatment in American TCs is recounted by Kaufman and De Leon (1975).

Even the early developments were the subjects of intensive evaluations. Evaluation researchers were reported by Curle (1947), Curle and Trist (1947), and Wilson, Curle, and Trist (1952). A reading finds this work still among quality examinations of the therapeutic community. These first reviews investigated the initial TC effects aimed at altering neurotic behaviors. There were soon explorations of other uses.

The basic TC premises were communicated to large numbers of the professional community Maxwell Jones (1952, 1953, 1962, 1968a, 1968b, 1976). It became part of American training in psychiatric texts (Kraft 1966). By this year 1980, its dissemination is international in scope crossing the boundaries of almost all continents. Utilization for client populations is equally broad embracing many aspects of mental health disorders, plus a variety of drug and alcohol addictions, and criminal justice problems. Hinshelwood and Manning (1979) provide an excellent update on conceptual and operational progress and is an indicator of the breadth of experience.

The evidence in support of TC effectiveness is mounting, yet there are still many areas to be explored. Whiteley (1979) suggests development needs in the area of mental health. Iverson and Wenger (1978-79) note that there are a range of research tasks in addiction incuding examination of the psychological/sociological principles, counter productive practices and cost efficiency. De Leon has continued to expand on client population definition and requests further work, (see e.g. De Leon, Rosenthal & Brodney 1971; De Leon, Skodol & Rosenthal, 1973; Wexler & De Leon, 1977 and De Leon & Koslowsky, 1978). Ziegenfuss (Note 1) would combine the work in a general movement toward comprehensive examination and refinement.

Although problem areas and study topics may differ, concensus on the need for continued development seems to be emerging. Should we not plan for and encourage the outcome? This paper presents a proposal for such a plan. Importantly, planning is viewed as action undertaken for the purpose of effecting change and includes both the definition of the change purpose and the design of actions for change (Ozbekhan, 1975).

A Proposal for Continued Therapeutic Community Development

It is sufficiently evident to researchers and clinicians in the field that the therapeutic community is not fully defined, developed, implemented or evaluated. To assure scientific efficiency and to enhance quality and quantity of progress a plan is required for organizing this work. To this end, a planning proposal for continued international development of the therapeutic community is offered.

Following the system planning model of Ackoff (1970), the plan proposal has five parts: ends, means, resources, implementation and control. With concern for both social and technical dimensions (Trist, 1963, 1973), they are:

Ends: specification of objectives and goals.

Means: selection of policies, programs, procedures, and practices by which objectives and goals are to be pursued.

Resources: determination of the types and amounts of resources required, how they are to be generated or acquired, and how they are to be allocated to activities.

Implementation: design of decision-making procedures and a way of organizing them so that the plan can be carried out.

Control: design of the procedure for anticipating or detecting errors in, or failures of the plan and for preventing or correcting them on a continuing basis.

Much of the plan design will not be new as it should occur inevitably in the world-wide development and acceptance of any product or service. The plan is designed to foster the conditions for renewed and collaborative work.

The following presents some suggestions for each of the five planning parts. A planning group is recommended as a mechanism — they would be expected to elaborate or alter what is here presented only as a starting point.

Ends

First, the ends of the plan are generally to continue the development of the therapeutic community across and within at least five topic areas: addictions; criminal justice; education; mental health and mental retardation; and business management and training. This purpose must be interpreted through a set of goal statements as follows:

Goals:

To increase the level and pace of international development of the therapeutic community through concept utilization and research.

To increase the clinical and organizational uses of the therapeutic community.

To increase the theoretical and empirical research on the therapeutic community.

These are to be accomplished through the following objectives:

Objectives:

To increase **communication** between therapeutic community practitioners and researchers in all countries and states.

To increase **coordination** of therapeutic community development efforts in both practice and research.

To increase **collaboration** on therapeutic community development projects in both practice and research.

These goals can be illustrated by example. In mental health (only one of the TC utilization areas) the TC is viewed as a first generation model of the theory and practice of psycho-social rehabilitation programs.[1] It is one of a few (or perhaps the only) serious competitors to the long established medical model (Blaney, 1975) which may be dying (Torrey, 1974). There is believed to be an idealized design for this model. The goal is to continue model development through a series of successively improving approximations to the ideal design.

Achievement of progress in successive approximations requires evaluation of all components of the mental health therapeutic communities through the comparisons of models in use (see e.g. Manning and Blake, 1979). Identification of some components appears in Table 1. Model refinement further necessitates a series of specific goals for individual development of each of the components (of course, constantly relating these parts to the whole model). For example, how well TC's manage patients rights has been questioned (Ziegenfuss and Gaughan-Fickes, 1976). But exploration of TC structure and process suggested

---

[1] The therapeutic community as a representative of the psychosocial school is in conflict with the medical model which may be referred to as a paradigm clash (Kuhn, 1962).

that it may be "the" model for implementing civil liberties of mental patients (Ziegenfuss, 1977). Through this continual examination process, an idealized model of the TC for mental health care will be created. For our plan we must keep in mind that mental health is only one area of work. Total planning goals apply both across and within topic areas, e.g. addictions, education and business management and training.

Means

Second, the plan requires a means of achieving this development. The overarching policy is one of uniting diverse TC efforts. Linking international TC scholars and practioners for joint endeavors enhances the quality of the development and the speed at which it progresses. Seven policy statements are relevant.

1. Establishment of an international community of TC practitioners and researchers will be encouraged.
2. Examination and re-examination of the theoretical and operational tenets of the TC will be encouraged.
3. International support for new or innovative TC operations will be developed.
4. Identification of research needs on a level which reflects TC breadth (e.g. multiple topics) and depth (e.g. TC structure and client characteristics) will be conducted.
5. Additional inter-country and intra-country communications on TC progress will be established.
6. Similar TC development efforts within and between countries will be linked.
7. New TC development efforts will be encouraged as team efforts.

Actions taken in support of these policies would lead to development progress in practice and research. The policies are consistent with the objectives of increased communication, coordination and collaboration.

Resources

To achieve development goals three types of resources will be required: people, money, and facilities. They are all critical for TC growth but human resources are first in importance.

The rationale for people support of collaborative development follows the notion that the whole is greater than the sum of its parts. As the TC's strength is based on the totality of the system greater than the individual components' sum, a community of researchers and practitioners working on development realizes the same state. A community collaborative development effort is consistent with both the philosophy of the TC and the sociology of knowledge finding that breakthroughs are increasingly more common from teams than from "lone wolf" investigators, particularly in interdiscipinary applied research, Ackoff (1962, 1974).

This viewpoint necessitates a linking of human resources. Practitioners and researchers must join on two levels: (1) within and between countries and (2) within and between TC topic areas (e.g. within addictions and between addictions and mental health). This social networking has already begun. The British, Netherlands, and American Associations of Therapeutic Communities have organized within countries and have initiated exchanges between country (the United Kingdom-Netherlands Conference 1979, Note 2 and the International TC Congresses 1973 to 1979 Note 3). Networking in topic areas, particularly between areas, has made limited progress.

Funding for the development effort must be generated by the people commitment. All TC researchers and practitioners must struggle individually for resources to keep service and research going. Joining forces will enhance both the power to make financial needs known and the capacity to initiate and complete TC projects on a high level, in turn generating more support (for example through research, Manning, 1979). The primary funding targets are government, foundation and private corporate and individual sources.

The final resource are facilities or centers. A quick extension of the development will require concentration of research and training at sites which have already developed credibility in their area. In mental health, work could center at the Henderson and Littlemore Hospitals, Oxford University and at the Albany Medical College hospital in America. Addictions, criminal justice and other topic areas would have their own bases.

With goals and policies outlined and resources needs suggested, we need to assemble them in an operational scheme.

Implementation

Development of the international effort will require five steps: (1) Formation of a Planning Committee; (2) Task and Project Definition; (3) Task Group Formation and Action Plans; (4) Overall and Individual

Funding; (5) Special and Regular Meetings to Review Progress. A group must be identified to initiate the steps. Given the purposes and history, the British Association of Therapeutic Communities would seem one logical choice to assume organizing responsibility.

To implement this plan we must first form a planning committee. The committee's responsibilities would include: (1) defining the scope and content of the effort; (2) setting policies and procedures; (3) developing Task Forces and Subcommittees as appropriate; (4) reviewing work reports and synthesizing recommendations into a plan; and (5) promoting and obtaining endorsement for the plan. Membership would be drawn from the British, Dutch, American and other TC associations, professional associations (e.g. psychiatry, psychology), colleges, and universities and individual TCs and researchers. The committee could be organized by using conferences already established such as the International Congress on Group Psychotherapy (Note 4), and could develop the NATO Scientific Seminar suggested by Whiteley (Note 5) and the British Association of Therapeutic Communities.

The second step would involve task and problem definition by the committee. Several questions might open the discussion:

1. What are the dominant TC practice/operations issues to be resolved?
2. What are the dominant research questions?
3. What is the availability and utilization of TC training?

TC Practice, Research and Training might be the three headings for development of detailed objectives. Table 1 provides a sample outline of subjects and topic areas which would map the work progress, of course with detailed subject points (Ziegenfuss, 1976, Note 1). A survey of TC practitioners might be used to identify and rank order topics for priority. When this was completed, Task Groups within and between countries could work on each of the areas. Three specific tasks could be considered as starting points:

1. Practice: development of an inventory of TC concept uses and client groups.
2. Research: development of a cross-cultural client characteristics study.
3. Training: development of a one week training program modeled on the American National Institute of Mental Health's staff college.

Table 1

SAMPLE DEVELOPMENT SUBJECTS BY TOPIC AREA*

Topic Areas Subjects	Mental Health & Mental Retardation	Criminal Justice	Education	Addictions	Business Management & Training
PRACTICE – history – structure & process – funding					
RESEARCH – client characteristics – evaluation – cross cultural differences – assumptions					
TRAINING – needs – models – availability					

*The intersecting points must be systematically addressed by existing and new development work.

Once tasks are defined funding is the third step. Government, foundations and private corporations/individuals support could be generated by the collaboration. A funding plan defining within-country and between-country responsibilities would be developed. Initially, a single grant proposal would be formulated to cover expenses of the focal planning effort.

Last, we must continue the efforts through progress reports at special and regular meetings. The International Congress of Therapeutic Communities, the UK-Netherlands Conference on TC's; the International Congress on Group Psychotherapy; and others could include sections which review planning and action steps. This new **International Journal of Therapeutic Communities** can be a vital communication mechanism.

Control

The plan must have an evaluation/control mechansim for determining its progress toward the goals. The steering committee could be that mechansim. Meeting twice a year, they would review information relative to the six stated goals as the following:

1. level and pace of TC development indicated by the frequency of publications, projects, and amounts of funding;
2. uses indicated by the number of new projects and use areas;
3. theoretical and empirical contributions indicated by the numbers and quality of journal articles and books;
4. communications indicated by the numbers of TC conferences, meetings, and public announcements;
5. coordination indicated by the numbers of cross references to similar projects in TC practice and research;
6. collaboration indicated by the number of joint projects and linked efforts.

These indicators merely illustrate the kinds of data that could be collected to monitor the effectiveness of the plan. In the event that the activities are not leading to goal achievement, the action plan would be modified as appropriate. That is, the plan is viewed as a dynamic document subject to constant revisions suggested by the evaluation/control group.

Summary

To continue the development of the therapeutic community, an international interdisciplinary effort must be initiated. Individual efforts while certainly contributory can be supported and enhanced by networks which represent the diversity of therapeutic community work in many disciplines, problem areas and countries.

This plan is in total quite ambitious. Yet we would regard success as development progress on each point, no matter the scale. Increased acceptance and utilization of the therapeutic community depends on the design and discovery of critical structure and process characteristics. We can best do that as collaborators. It is, after all, what the therapeutic community is about! Collaborative international development will demonstrate that we developers also feel that a whole is greater than the sum of the parts.

Notes

1. Ziegenfuss, J.T. *The therapeutic community from 1970-75: A Review and A Proposal for Continued Development,* Presented at United Kingdom-Netherlands Workshop of Therapeutic Communities, Cumberland Lodge, Windsor, England, September 1978.
2. United Kingdom — Netherlands Conference on Therapeutic Communities Cumberland Lodge 1978. Sponsored by the British and Dutch Assns of Therapeutic Communities.
3. International Congress on Therapeutic Communities. New York, 1979 Meeting.
4. International Congress of Group Psychotherapy. Copenhagen, Denmark. 1980 Meeting.
5. Whiteley, J. Proposal for a North Atlantic Treaty Organization (NATO) Scientific Seminar on Therapeutic Communities. Sponsor British Assn of TCs. 1978.

BIBLIOGRAPHY

Abruzzi, W. (1979). The Failure of Therapeutic Communities, Drug Treatment and Rehabilitation Programs. *International Journal of Addiction*, 14, pp. 1023-1030.

Ackoff, R.L. (1962). *Scientific Method*. New York: Wiley.

Ackoff, R.L. (1970). *A Concept of Corporate Planning*. New York: Wiley.

Ackoff, R.L. (1974). *Redesigning the Future*. New York: Wiley.

Ackoff, R.L. & Emery, F.E. (1972). *On Purposeful Systems*. Chicago: Aldine-Antherton.

Almond, R. (1974). *The Healing Community: Dynamics of the Therapeutic Milieu*. New York: Jason Aronson, p. 327.

Anon, R.S. (1978, November). The Synanon Horrors. *New Times, 11*, pp. 28-50.

Anonymous (1939). *Alcoholics Anonymous*. New York: Alcoholics Anonymous World Service.

Anonymous (1952). *Twelve Steps and Twelve Traditions*. New York: Alcoholics Anonymous World Service.

Anscombe, F.J. & Tukey, J.W. (1963). The Examination and Analysis of Residuals. *Technometrics, 5*, pp. 141-61.

Antze, P. (1979). Role of Ideologies in Peer Psychotherapy Groups. In M. Lieberman & L.D. Borman (Eds.), *Self-Help Groups for Coping With Crisis*. San Francisco: Jossey-Bass.

Arn, I. (1975). Daytop — A Drug-Free Addict Care Programme. *Lakartidningen, 72*, pp. 3013-3016.

Aron, W.S. & Daily, D. (1974). Camarillo — Short and Long-Term Therapeutic Communities: A Follow-up and Cost Effectiveness Comparison. *International Journal of Addiction, 9*, pp. 619-636.

Aron, W.S. & Daily, D.W. (1976). Graduates and Splittees from Therapeutic Community Drug Treatment Programs: A Comparison. *International Journal of Addictions, 11*, pp. 1-18.

Asher, H.B. (1976). *Causal Modeling*. Beverly, CA: Sage Publications.

Azima, F.C. (1984, April 24). An Examination of Leadership Patterns in Cults. *Workshop VIIIth International Congress of Group Psychotherapy*. Mexico City, Mexico.

Bale, R.N. (1979). Outcome Research in Therapeutic Communities for Drug Abusers: A Critical Review 1963-1975. *The International Journal of the Addictions, 14*, pp. 1053-1074.

Bale, R. & Cabrera, S. (1977). Follow-up Evaluation of Drug Abuse Treatment. *American Journal of Drug Alcohol Abuse, 4*(2), pp. 233-249.

249

Bale R.N., Van Stone, W.W., Kuldau, J.M., Engelsing, T.M.J., Elashoff, R.M. & Zarcone, V.P., Jr. (1980). Therapeutic Communities vs. Methadone Maintenance. *Archives of General Psychiatry, 37,* pp. 179-193.

Bale, R.N., Van Stone, W.W., Kuldau, J.M., Engelsing, T.M. & Zarcone, V.P. (1973). Methadone Treatment vs. Therapeutic Communities: Preliminary Results of a Randomised Study on Progress. *National Conference on Methadone Treatment Proceedings, 2,* pp. 1027-1034.

Barnard, C.I. (1938). *The Functions of an Executive.* Cambridge: Harvard University Press, p. 163.

Barr H., Cohen A. (1979): *The Problem-Drinking Drug Addict.* (DHEW Publication No. (ADM) 79-893). National Institute on Drug Abuse, Services Research Report.

Barr, H.L., Ottenberg, D.J. & Rosen, A. (1972). Two Year Follow-up Study of 724 Drug Addicts and Alcoholics Treated Together in an Abstinence Therapeutic Community. Presented at the National Conference on Methadone Treatment: Washington, D.C.

Bassin, A.(1977). The Miracle of the TC.: From Birth to Post-Partum Insanity to Full Recovery. In P. Vamos & J.E. Brown (Eds.), *Proceedings of the 2nd World Conference of Therapeutic Communities* (p. 14). Montreal, Canada: Portage Press.

Bassin, A., Bratter, T.C. & Ranchin, R.L. (1976). *The Reality Therapy Reader.* New York: Harper & Row Publication.

Becker, H.S. (1960). Notes on the Concept of Commitment. *American Journal of Sociology, 66,* pp. 32-40.

Becker, H.S. (1963). *Outsiders.* New York: Free Press.

Bejerot, N. (1972). A Theory of Addiction as an Artifically Induced Drive. *American Journal of Psychiatry, 7,* pp. 842-46.

Bentham, J. (1914). *Theory of Legislation.* In C.M. Atrinson (Trans.), (Vol. 1). Oxford: Claredon Press. pp. 1-5, (translated by C.M. Atkison).

Biase, D.V. (1982). Daytop Miniversity: College Training Within a Therapeutic Community (PB 82-172537). Springfield, VA: U.S. Department of Commerce, National Technical Information Service.

Biase, D.V. (1972). Phoenix Houses: Therapeutic Communities for Drug Addicts. In W. Krup (Ed.), *Drug Abuse, Current Concepts and Research.* Springfield IL: Charles C Thomas.

Biase, D.V. (1974). Phoenix Houses: Therapeutic Communities for Drug Addicts. In G. De Leon (Ed.), *Phoenix House: Studies in a Therapeutic Community (1968-73).* New York: MSS Information Corporation.

Biase, D.V. (1983). The College Program at Daytop New York. *7th World Conference on Therapeutic Communities,* Chicago.

Biase, D.V. & De Leon, G. (1969). The Encounter Group: Measurement of Some Affect Changes. *Proceedings, 77th American Psychological Association.* Washington, D.C.

Blaney, P.H. (1975). Implications of the Medical Model and its Alternatives. *American Journal Psychiatry, 9,* p. 132.

Blum, R.H. (1969). Normal Drug use. In Blum and Associates (Eds.), *Society and Drugs.* San Francisco: Jossey-Bass.

Boruch, R.F. & Gomez, H. (1977). Sensitivity, Bias and Theory in Impact Evaluation. *Professional Psychology, 8,* pp. 411-434.

Bowes, R. (1974). The Industry as Pusher. *Journal of Drug Issues, 4*, pp. 138-242.

Bracy, S.A. & Simpson, D.D. (1982-83). Status of Opioid Addicts 5 Years After Admission to Drug Abuse Treatment. *American Journal of Drug and Alcohol Abuse, 9*(2), pp. 115-127.

Braginsky, D.D. (1975). The Mentally Ill, the Alcoholic, the Drug Addict: Misfits All. In D.J. Ottenberg & E.L. Carpey (Eds.), *Proceedings of the 7th Annual Eagleville Conference,* Rockville, MD. Alcohol, Drug Abuse, and Mental Health Administration, pp. 105-112.

Braginsky, D.D. & Braginsky, B.M. (1973, December). Psychologists: High Priests of the Middle Class. *Psychology Today, 15,* pp. 18-20, 138-139, 142.

Bray, R.M., Hubbard, R.L., Rachal, J.V., Cavanaugh, E.R., Craddock, S.G., Collins, J.J., Schlenger, W.E. & Allison, M. (1981). Summary and Implications: Client Characteristics, Behaviors and In-Treatment Outcomes, 1979, TOPS Admission Cohort. Research Triangle Institute, North Carolina.

Bratter, T.E. (1977). Confrontation Groups: The Therapeutic Community's Gift to Psychotherapy. In P. Vamos & J.J. Delvin (Eds.), *The Proceedings of the First World Conference on Therapeutic Communities* (pp. 164-176). Montreal, Canada: The Portage Press.

Bratter, T.E. (1977b). Varfor Blir Ungdomar Drogmissbrukare? *Socionom Forbundents, 3,* pp. 10-17.

Bratter, T.E. (1978). The Four 'R's' of the American Self-Help Therapeutic Community: Rebirth, Responsibility, Reality, and Respect. In J. Corelli, I. Bonfiglio, T Pediconi & M. Colloumb (Eds.), *Preceedings of the Third World Conference of Therapeutic Communities.* (pp. 434-448). Rome, Italy: International Council of Alcohol and Addictions Press.

Bratter, T.E. (1980. Les Communates Therapeutiques Aux Etats Unis: Une Approache Nouvelle et Humaniste de la Toxicomanie. *Transitions: Revenue de l'Innovation Psychiatrique et Sociale, 3,* pp. 86-98.

Bratter, T.E. (in press). Group Psychotherapy with Alcoholically and Drug Addicted Adolescents: Special Clinical Concerns. In F.C. Azima & L.H. Richmond (Eds.), *Adolescent Group Psychotherapy.* New York: International Universities Press.

Bratter, T.E., Collabolletta, E.A., Fossbender, A.J., Gauya, D.A., Pennacchia, M.C. & Rubel, J.R. (in press). The American Self-Help Therapeutic Community: A Pragmatic Treatment Approach for Addicted Character-Disordered Individuals. In T.E. Bratter & G. Forrest (Eds.), *The Management of Alcoholics and Substance Abusers.* New York: Free Press.

Bratter, T.E. & Kooyman, M. (1980). A Structured Environment for Heroin Addicts: The Experiences of A Community-Based American Methadone Clinic and A Residential Dutch Therapeutic Community. *The International Journal of Social Psychiatry, 19,* pp. 189-203.

Brecher, E.M. (1972). *Licit and Illicit Drugs.* Boston: Little, Brown.

Bredemeier, H.C. (1978). *Evaluations.* Unpublished manuscript, Rutgers University.

Bredemeier, H.C. (1979). *Locating the Meaning of Things.* Unpublished manuscript, Rutgers University.

Bridger, H. (1946). The northfield experiment. *Bulletin of the Menninger Clinic, 10,* p. 3.

252   *Therapeutic Communities for Addictions*

Brill, L. & Lieberman, L. (1969). *Authority and Addiction*. Boston: Little Brown, pp. 60, 15.

Campbell, D.T. & Stanley, J.C. (1963). *Experimental and Quasi-Experimental Designs for Research*. Chicago: Rand McNally.

Carden, M.C. (1969). *Onedia: Utopian Community to Modern Corporation*. Baltimore: Johns Hopkins Press.

Carlson, K. (1976). Heroin, Hassle and Treatment: The Importance of Perceptual Differences. *Addictive Diseases, 2*(4), pp. 569-584.

Carroll, J.F.X. (1975). Mental Illness and Disease: Outmoded Concepts in Alcohol and Drug Rehabilitation. *Community Mental Health Journal, 2*, pp. 418-429.

Carroll, J.F.X. (1978, Summer). Mental Illness and Addiction: Perspectives Which Overemphasize Differences and Undervalue Commonalities. *Contemporary Drug Problems*, pp. 117-231.

Carroll, J.F.X. (1979, Fall). Do Contemporary Drug/Alcohol Treatment Strategies Create A Basic Conflict Between Ethical Concerns and Treatment Effectiveness? *Contemporary Drug Problems*, pp. 389-404.

Carroll, J.F.X., Klein, M.I. & Santo, Y. (1978). Comparisons of the Similarities and Differences in the Self-Concepts of Male Alcoholics and Addicts. *Journal of Consulting and Clinical Psychology, 46*, pp. 575-576.

Casriel, D. (1966). *So Fair A House: The Story of Synanon*. New York: Prentice Hall.

Casriel, D. (1972). *A Scream Away from Happiness*. New York: Grosset & Dunlop.

Catalano, R.F., Hawkins, J.D. & Hall, J.A. (1983). *Preventing Relapse Among Former Substance Abusers*. University of Washington, Center for Social Welfare, Research.

Chambers, C.D. & Inciardi, J.A. (1974). Three Years After the Split. In E. Senay & V. Shorty (Eds.), *Developments in the Field of Drug Abuse*. Cambridge: Schenkman.

Chein, I., Gerard, D.L., Lee, R.S. & Rosenfeld, E. (1964). *The Road to H*. New York: Basic Books.

Christ, J. (1975). Contrasting the Charismatic and Reflective Leader. In Z.A. Liff (Ed.), *The Leader in the Group*. New York: Jason Aronson, p. 104.

Clausen, J.A. (1957). Social Patterns, Personality, and Adolescent Drug Use. In A.H. Leighton et al. (Eds.), *Exploration in Social Psychiatry*. New York: Basic Books.

Cline, S. & Goldberg, P. (1976). *Government Response to Drug Abuse: The 1977 Budget*. Washington, D.C.: Drug Abuse Council.

Cohen, J. & Cohen P. (1975). *Applied Multiple Regression/Correlation Analysis for the Behavioral Sciences*. Hillsdale, NJ: John Wiley.

Collins, B.E. & Hoyt, M.F. (1972). Personal Responsibility for Consequences: An Integration and Extension of the "Forced Compliance Literature." *Journal of Experimental Social Psychology, 8*, pp. 558-73.

Condelli, W.S. (1976). *Competing Models of Drug Use*. Unpublished manuscript, Rutgers University.

Condelli, W.S. (1983). External Pressure and Retention in Therapeutic Communities. *International Journal of Therapeutic Communities*.

Coombs, R.H. (1981). Back on the Streets: Therapeutic Communities' Impact Upon Drug Users. *American Journal of Drug and Alcohol Abuse, 8,*(2), pp. 185-201.

Curle, A. (1946). Transitional Communities and Social Re-Connection, Part II. *Human Relations, 1*, p. 1.

Curle, A. & Trist, E.L. (1947). Transitional Communities and Social Re-Connection, Part II. *Human Relations, 1,* p. 1.

Deitch, D.A. (1972). Treatment of Drug Abuse in the Therapeutic Community: Historical Influences, Current Considerations, and Future Outlooks. *National Commission on Marihuana and Drug Abuse, IV,* pp. 158-75.

Deitch, D. (1983). Codification. In M. Darcy (Ed.), *Proceedings of the 7th World Conference of Therapeutic Communities* (p. 176). Chicago: Gateway Press.

Deitch, D. & Zweben, J.E. (1979). Synanon: A Pioneering Response to Drug Abuse Treatment and A Signal for Caution. In S. Halpern & B. Levine (Eds.), *Proceedings of the Fourth International Conference of Therapeutic Communities* (pp. 57-70). New York: Daytop Village Press.

D'Entreves, A.P. (1951). *Natural Law.* London: Hutchinson's University Library, p. 57.

DeBruce, D.J. (1975). Good but   , The Story of Becoming A Therapist at Eagleville Hospital. In D.J. Ottenberg & E.L. Carpey (Eds.), *Proceedings of the 7th Annual Eagleville Conference* (pp. 151-156). Rockville, MD, Alcohol, Drug Abuse, and Mental Health Administration.

De Leon, G. (1974). (Editor). *Phoenix House: Studies in a Therapeutic Community (1968-1973).* New York: MSS Press.

De Leon, G. (1976) *Psychologic and Socio-Demographic Profiles.* Final Report of Phoenix House Project Activities, Grant No. DA-00831. Rockville, MD: National Institute on Drug Abuse.

De Leon, G. (1979). People and data systems. *Management Information Systems in the Drug Field.* Services Research Series. (Eds). G. Beschner & C. D'Amanda Rockville, MD: National Institute on Drug Abuse. DHHS # (ADM)79-836

De Leon, G. (1980a). *Therapeutic Communities: Training Self-Evaluation.* Final Report of Project Activities. Grant No. 1-H81-DA-01976. Rockville, MD: National Institute on Drug Abuse.

De Leon, G. (1980b). Evaluating Effectiveness: Proving Treatment Influence May Be A Non-Issue. Paper presented National Alcohol and Drug Conference, Washington, D.C.

De Leon, G. (1981). The Role of Rehabilitation. In C.G. Nahas & H.C. Frick (Eds.), *Drug Abuse in the Modern World: A Perspective for the Eighties.* New York: Pergamon Press.

De Leon, G. (1983a). *The TC: Predicting Retention and Follow-up Status.* Final Report of Project Activities. Grant No. 1-R01-DA 02741-01A1. Rockville, MD: National Institute on Drug Abuse.

De Leon, G. (1983b). The next therapeutic community: Autocracy, and other notes toward integrating old and new therapeutic communities. *International Journal of Therapeutic Communities, 4,* p. 249-261.

De Leon, G. (1984a). *The Therapeutic Community: Study of Effectivenss.* Treatment Research Monograph Series. Rockville, MD: National Institute on Drug Abuse, DHHS Pub. No.(ADM)84-1286.

De Leon, G. (1984b). Program Based Evaluation Research in TCs. In F. Tims & J. Ludford (Eds.), *Drug Abuse Treatment Evaluation: Strategies, Progress, and Prospects.* Research Analysis and Utilization System (RAUS) Monograph Series. Rockville, MD: National Institute on Drug Abuse. DHHS Pub. No.(ADM)84-1329, pp. 69-87.

De Leon, G. (1984c). *Treatment Process for Favorable Outcomes.* Paper presented American Psychological Association, Toronto, Canada.

De Leon, G. (1985). The therapeutic community: Status and evolution. *International Journal of the Addictions.* In press.

De Leon, G. & Andrews, M. (1978). Therapeutic community dropouts 5 years later: Preliminary findings on self reported status. In Smith (Ed.), *A Multi-Cultural View of Drug Abuse: Proceedings of the National Drug Abuse Conference.* Cambridge, MA: Schenkman, pp. 369-378.

De Leon, G. & Beschner, G. (1977). *The Therapeutic Community. Proceedings of Therapeutic Communities of America Planning Conference.* Rockville, MD: National Institute on Drug Abuse.

De Leon, G. & Biase, D.V. (1975). The encounter group: Measurement of systolic blood pressure. *Psychological Reports, 37,* pp. 439-445.

De Leon, G. & Jainchill, N. (1981-82). Male and female drug abusers: Social and psychological status 2 years after treatment in a therapeutic community. *American Journal of Drug & Alcohol Abuse. 8(4),* pp. 465-497.

De Leon, G. & Koslowsky, M.S. (1978). Therapeutic community dropouts: A global index of success and psychological status five years after treatment. *Eastern Psychological Association Conference.* Washington, D.C.

De Leon, G. & Rosenthal, M.S. (1979). Therapeutic communities. In R. DuPont, A. Goldstein & J. O'Donnell (Eds.), *Handbook on Drug Abuse.* Rockville, MD: National Institute on Drug Abuse.

De Leon, G. & Schwartz, S. (1984). The therapeutic community: What are the retention rates? *American Journal of Drug & Alcohol Abuse. 10(2),* 267-284.

De Leon, G. & Wexler, H. (1973). Heroin addiction: Its relation to sexual experience. Journal of Abnormal Psychology. 81, pp. 36-38.

De Leon, G., Andrews, M., Wexler, H., Jaffe, J. & Rosenthal, M.S. (1979). Therapeutic community dropouts: Criminal behavior five years after treatment. *American Journal of Drug and Alcohol Abuse. 6* pp. 253-271.

De Leon, G., Holland, S. & Rosenthal, M.S. (1972). Phoenix House: Criminal activity of dropouts. *Journal of the American Medical Association, 222,* pp. 686-689.

De Leon, G., Rosenthal, M. & Brodney, K. (1971). Therapeutic community for drug addicts. Long-term measurement of emotional changes. *Psychological Reports, 29,* pp. 595-600.

De Leon, G., Skodol, A. & Rosenthal, M.S. (1973). The Phoenix Therapeutic Community for drug addicts: Changes in psychopathological signs. *Archives of General Psychiatry, 28,* pp. 131-135.

De Leon, G., Wexler, H.K. & Jainchill, N. (1982). The therapeutic community: Success & improvement rates 5 years after treatment. *International Journal of the Addictions, 17,* pp. 703-747.

De Leon, G., Wexler, H.K., Schwartz, S., and Jainchill, N. (1980). *Therapeutic Communities for Drug Abusers: Studies of the Treatment Environment.* Paper presented to the American Psychological Asociation, Toronto, Canada.

De Long, J.V. (1972). The Drugs and Their Effects. In P.M. Wald & P.B. Hutt

(Eds.), *Dealing With Drug Abuse.* New York: Praeger.

Des Jarlais, D.; Joseph, H., & Dole, V. (1981). Long-term outcomes after termination from methadone maintenance treatment. *Annals of New York Academy of Science. 362*, 231-238.

Des Jarlais, D.C., Knott, A., Savarese, J. & Bersamin, J. (1976). Rules and Rule Breaking in A Therapeutic Community. *Addictive Diseases: An International Journal*, *2*, pp. 627-641.

Dies, R.R. & Hess, A.K. (1971). An Experimental Investigation of Cohesiveness in Marathon and Conventional Group Therapy. *Journal of Abnormal and Social Psychology, 77*, pp. 258-62.

Dole, V.P. & Nyswander, M.E. (1967). Heroin Addiction — A Metabolic Disease. *Archives of Internal Medicine, 120*, pp. 19-24.

Dominicus, R.D. (1974). Therapeutic Community for Alcoholics: Experience with A Milieu Therapy Department of A Psychiatric Hospital. *Nervenarzt, 45*, pp. 200-206.

Donnenberg, D. (1978). Art Therapy in A Drug Community. *Confinia Psychiatrica, 21*, pp. 37-44.

Duster, T. (1970). *The Legislation of Morality: Laws, Drugs, and Moral Judgment.* New York: Free Press.

Edmondson, W.R. (1972). Long-Term Rehabilitation of the Drug Dependent Person: The Odyssey House Method. *Journal of the National Medical Association, 64*, pp. 502-504.

Eisman, B. (1959). Some Operational Measures of Cohesiveness and Their Correlations. *Human Relations, 12*, pp. 183-89.

Emerson, R.W. (1913). *Essays 1st and 2nd Series.* London: Dent.

Emrick, C.D. & Hansen, J. (1983). Assertions Regarding Effectiveness of Treatment Alcoholism: Fact or Fantasy? *American Psychologist, 38,* pp. 1078-1088.

Etzioni, A. (1964). Modern Organizations, Englewood Cloffs, deutsch: Soziologie der Organisationen, Juventa, Munchen, 1967.

Etzioni, A. (1961). Ed.: A Basis for Comparative Analysis of Complex Organizations, Glencoe Free Press.

Fischmann, V.S. (1968). Drug Addicts in A Therapeutic Community: Outline on the Californian Rehabilitation Centre Programme, Corona. *Psychotherapy & Psychosomatics, 16*, pp. 109-118.

Fitts, W.H. (1972). *The Self Concept and Psychopathology.* Monograph IV, Nashville, TN: Counselor Recordings and Tests.

Fitts, W.H. & Hamner, W.T. (1969). *The Self Concept and Delinquency.* Monography I, Nashville, TN: Counselor Recordings and Tests.

Foureman, W.C., Parks, R. & Gardin, T.H. (1981). The MMPI as A Predictor of Retention in A Therapeutic Community for Heroin Addicts. *International Journal of Addiction, 16*, pp. 893-903.

Frank, J. (1961). *Persuasion and Healing: A Comparative Study of Psychotherapy.* Baltimore: Johns Hopkins Press.

Freud, S. (1962). *Civilization and Its Discontents.* New York: W.W. Norton.

Freudenberger, H.J. (1974). How We Can Right What's Wrong With Our Therapeutic Communities. *Journal of Drug Issues, 4*, pp. 251-259.

Freudenberger, H.J. (1976). Proceedings: The Therapeutic Community Revisited. *American Journal of Drug Alcohol Abuse, 3*, pp. 33-49.

Freudenberger, H.J. (1980). The Issues of Re-entry for the Resident and Staff in Therapeutic Communities. *Journal of Psychedelic Drugs, 12,* pp. 65-69.

Fromm, E. (1941). *Escape From Freedom.* New York: Rinehart, p. 168.

Fromm, E. (1955). *The Sane Society.* New York: Rinehart, p. 237.

Fromm, E. (1973). *The Anatomy of Human Destructiveness.* New York: Holt, Rinehart and Winston, p. 38.

Galanter, M. (1982). Charismatic Religious Sects and Psychiatry: An Overview. *American Journal of Psychiatry, 139,* pp. 1539-1547.

Glaser, F.B. (1974). some Historical Aspects of the Drug-Free Therapeutic Community. *American Journal of Drug Alcohol Abuse, 1.* pp. 37-52.

Glaser, F.B. (1974). Splitting: Attrition from A Drug-Free Therapeutic Community. *American Journal of Drug Alcohol Abuse, 1,* pp. 329-348.

Glaser, F.B. (1981). The Origins of the Drug-Free Therapeutic Community. *British Journal of Addiction, 76,* pp. 13-25.

Glasscote, R.M., Sussex, J.N., Ball, J. & Brill, L. (1972). *The Treatment of Drug Abuse.* Washington, D.C.: American Psychological Association.

Glasscote, R.M., Sussex, J.N., Jaffe, J., u.a., (1972). *The Treatment of Drug Abuse Programs, Problems, Prospects.* Washington, Joint Information Service.

Goffman, E. (1961). *Asylums.* Garden City, NY: Doubleday.

Golding, W.G. (1962). *Lord of the Flies.* New York: Coward-McCann.

Goldman, B. (1958). *Group Cohesiveness.* Chicago: Psychometric Affiliates.

Goldschmidt, P.G. (1976). A Cost-Effectiveness Model for Evaluating Health Care Programmes: Application to Drug Abuse Treatment. *Inquiry, 13,* pp. 29-47.

Goldstein, A. et al. (1968). *Principles of Drug Action.* New York: Harper & Row.

Goode, E. (1972). *Drugs in American Society.* New York: Knopf.

Goode, E. (1973). The Drug Pehnomenon: Social Aspects of Drug Taking. Indianapolis, IN: Bobbs-Merril.

Grossman, G. (1973). A Methadone Therapeutic Community: A Supplement to an Ambulatory Methadone Maintenance Unit. *National Conference on Methadone Treatment Proceedings, 1,* pp. 622-627.

Hagstrom, W.O. & Selvin, H.C. (1965). Two Dimensions of Cohesiveness in Small Groups. *Sociometry, 28,* pp. 30-43.

Hare, A.P. (1962). *Handbook of Small Group Research.* New York: Free Press, pp. 309, 318.

Harris, R., Linn, M.W. & Pratt, T.C. (1980). A Comparison of Drop-outs and Disciplinary Discharges from A Therapeutic Community. *International Journal of Addiction, 15,* pp. 749-756.

Hart, L. (1972). Milieu Management for Drug Addicts: Extended Drug Subculture or Rehabilitation? *British Journal of Addiction, 67,* pp. 297-301.

Hart, L. (1973). Attitudes Toward Drug Abuse Among Residents in A Therapeutic Community. *International Journal of Addiction, 8,* pp. 809-820.

Hart, L. (1974). Attitudes Towards Drug Abuse: Therapeutic Community (Concept) Residents vs. Methadone Patients. *British Journal of Addiction, 69,* pp. 375-379.

Harvey, R.H. (1949). *Robert Owens.* Berkeley: University of California Press.

Hasday, J.D. & Karch, F.E. (1981). Benzodiazepine Prescribing in A Family Medicine Center. *JAMA, 246,* pp. 1321-1325.

Hawkins, J.D. (1979). Reintegrating Street Drug Abusers. In B.S. Brown (Ed.), *Addicts and Aftercare.* Beverly Hills: Sage.

Hawkins, J.D. (1979). Some Suggestions for Self-Help Approaches with Street Drug Abusers. *Journal of Psychedelic Drugs, 12,* pp. 131-137.

Hawkins, J.D. & Wacker, N. (1983). Verbal Performances and Addict Conversion: An Interactionist Perspective on Therapeutic Communities. *Journal of Drug Issues, 13,* pp. 281-298.

Hegel, G. (1942). *Philosophy of the Right.* In T.M. Knox (Trans.), Oxford, England: Clarendon Press, pp. 155-156.

Heise, D.R. (1970). Semantic Differential and Attitude Research. In G.F. Summers (Ed.), *Attitude Measurement.* Chicago: Rand McNally.

Helmer, J. (1975). *Drugs and Minority Oppression.* New York: Seabury Press.

Henrich, G., de Jong, R., Mai, R. & Revenstorf, D. (1979). Aspekte des therapeutischen Klimas — Entwicklung eines Fragebogens. *Zeitung fur klinische Psychologie,* Vol. 8, pp. 41-55.

Herrera, J.J., Espinosa, N. & Cortopassi, L.O. (1969). The Therapeutic Community in Psychiatry. *Actas Luso Esp Neurol Psiquiatr 28,* pp. 100-116.

Hinds, W.A. (1878). *American Communities: Brief Sketches of Economy, Zoar, Bethel, Aurora, Icari, The Shakers, Oneida, Wallingford & The Brotherhood of New Life.* Oneida: Office of the American Socialist.

Hinshelwood, R.D. & Manning, N. (Eds.) (1979). *Therapeutic Communities.* London: Routledge & Kegan Paul.

Hobbes, T. (1904). *Leviathan.* Cambridge, England: Cambridge University Press, pp. 80-87.

Holland, S. (1978). Gateway Houses: Effectiveness of Treatment on Criminal Behaviour. *International Journal of Addiction, 13,* pp. 369-381.

Holland, S. (1981). *Drug Treatment Effectiveness: Using Multiple Data Probes to Strengthen Causal Inference.* Chicago, IL: Gateway Foundation.

Holland, S. (1982). *Residential Drug Free Programs for Substance Abusers: The Effect of Planned Duration on Treatment.* Chicago, IL: Gateway Foundation.

Hollidge, C. (1980). Psychodynamic Aspects of the Addicted Personality and Their Treatment in the Therapeutic Community. In Readings "Congresboek 5e Werelfkonferentie van therapeutische gemeenschappen," Samsom Sijthoff, Alphen aan de Rijn, pp. 61-86.

Homans, G.C. (1950). *The Human Group.* New York: Harcourt, Brace & World, Inc., pp. 419-420.

Homans, G.C. (1961). *Social Behavior: Its Elementary Forms.* New York: Harcourt, Brace & World, Inc., p. 294.

Hooker, C. (1976). Learned Helplessness. *Social Work, 21,* p. 194.

Horn, F. (1978). Encounter Group Therapy in A TC: Leaders and Casualties. In P. Vamos & J.E. Brown (Eds.), *Proceedings of the 2nd World Conference on Therapeutic Communities* (pp. 149-153). Montreal, Canada: Portage Press.

Huling, M. (1975). A Professional's View of Drug Abuse. In R.H. Coombs (ED.), *Junkies and Straights.* Lexington, MA: Lexington Books.

Huey, F.L. (1971). In A Therapeutic Community. *American Journal of Nursing, 71,* pp. 926-933.

Hunter, F. (1953). *Community Power Structure: A Study of Decision Makers.* Chapel Hill: University of North Carolina Press, pp. 2-3.

Isbell, H. (1966). Medical Aspects of Opiate Addiction. In J. O'Donnell & J.C. Ball (Eds.), *Narcotic Addiction.* New York: Harper & Row.

Iverson, D.C. & Wenger, S.S. (1978-1979). Therapeutic Communities: Treatment Practices in View of Drug Dependency Theory. *Drug Forum, 7,* p. 1.

Jackson, D.N. (1970). A Sequential System for Personality Scale Development. In C.D. Spielberger (Ed.), *Current Topics in Clinical and Community Psychology, 2,* New York: Academic Press.

Joe, G.W., & Chastain, R.L. (1984). Onset, Continuation, and Termination of Heroin Addiction. In *Heroin Addiction: 12-Year Posttreatment Follow-up Outcomes.* Symposium conducted at the meeting of the Southwestern Psychological Association, New Orleans.

Joe, G.W. & Simpson, D.D. (1976). Relationship of Patient Characteristics to Tenure. In S.B. Sells & D.D. Simpson (Eds.), *Studies in the Effectiveness of Treatment of Drug Abuse.* Cambridge, MA: Ballinger.

Johnson, G. (1976, Summer). Conversion as Cure: The Therapeutic Community and the Prof. Ex-addict. *Contemporary Drug Problem,* pp. 187-205.

Johnston, L.D., Nurco, D.N. & Robins, L.N. (1977). *Conducting Follow-up-Research on Drug Treatment Programs.* Rockville, NIDA.

Jones, M. (1952). *Social Psychiatry: The Therapeutic Community.* London: Tavistock Publications.

Jones, M. (1953). *The Therapeutic Community — A New Treatment Method in Psychiatry.* New York: Basic Books.

Jones, M. (1962). *Social Psychiatry in the Community in Hospitals and in Prisons.* Springfield, IL: Charles C Thomas.

Jones, M. (1968). *Beyond the Therapeutic Community — Social Learning and Social Psychiatry.* New Haven: Yale University Press.

Jones, M. (1968b). *Social Psychiatry in Practice.* Harmondsworth: Penguin.

Jones, M. (1976). *Maturation of the Therapeutic Community.* New York: Human Sciences Press.

Jones, M. (1978). Therapeutic Communities: Old and New. *Addiction Therapist, 3,* pp. 2-9.

Jones, M. (1979). Therapeutic Communities: Old and New. *American Journal of Drug Alcohol Abuse, 6*(2), pp. 137-149.

Jones, M. (1979). Therapeutic Communities: Old and New. *American Journal of Drug Alcohol Abuse, 69,* pp. 137-149.

Jongsma, T. (1980). What is Therapeutic in the Therapeutic Community? In: *Readings of the Fifth World Conference of Therapeutic Communities,* Noordwijkerhout, pp. 115-165, Samsom Sijthoff, Alphen aan de Rijn.

Jorstad, J. (1971). Young People with Drug Abuse Treated in A Therapeutic Community within A Psychiatric Hospital: Preliminary Experiences from Dikemark Hospital, Lien Department. *Tidsskr Nor Laegenforen, 91,* pp. 1367-1373.

Kandel, D.B. (1978). *Longitudinal Research on Drug Use.* New York: Wiley.

Kantor, R.M. (1968). Commitment and Social Organization: A Study of Commitment Mechanisms in Utopian Communities. *American Sociological Review, 33,* pp.
499-517.

Kaplan, E.H. & Weider, H. (1974). *Drugs Don't Take People, People Take Drugs.* Se-
caucus, NJ: Lyle Stuart.

Kaufman, E. (1979). The Therapeutic Community and Methadone: A Way of
Achieving Abstinence. *International Journal of Addiction, 14,* pp. 83-97.

Kaufman, E. & De Leon, G. (1978). The Therapeutic Community: A Treatment
Approach for Drug Abusers. Chapter 8: In A. Schecter (Ed.), *Treatment Aspects of
Drug Dependence.* Florida: CRC Press

Kaufman, E. & Kaufman, P.N. (1979). *Family Therapy of Drug and Alcohol Abuse.* New
York: Gardener Press.

Kemp, C.G. (1964). Differing Assumptions in Authoritarian, Democratic, and
Group-Centered Leadership. In C.G. Kemp (Ed.), *Perspectives on the Group Process:
A Foundation for Counseling with Groups.* Boston: Houghton Mifflin Company, p.
223.

Kennard, D. & Wilson, S. (1979). The Modification of Personality Disturbance in A
Therapeutic community for Drug Abusers. *British Journal of Medical Psychology, 52,*
pp. 215-221.

Kiev, A. (1964). *Magic, Faith, and Healing: Studies in Primitive Psychiatry Today.* New
York: The Free Press.

King, R. (1972). *The Drug Hangup: America's Fifty-Year Folloy.* New York: W.W. Norton.

Kittrie, N.K. (1971). *The Right to be Different: Deviance of Enforced Therapy.* Baltimore:
John Hopkins Press.

Kooyman, M. (1975). From Chaos to A Structured Therapeutic Community: Treatment Program on Emiliehoeve, A Farm for Young Addicts. *Bulletin on Narcotics,*
Vol. XXVII, *1,* pp. 19-26.

Kooyman, M. (1978). The History of the Therapeutic Community Movement in
Europe. *Proceedings of the 2nd World Conference of Therapeutic Community* (special edi-
tion 3, pp. 29-33). Montreal: The Addiction Therapist.

Kooyman, M. (1979). Pathology in the Therapeutic Community: The Role of the
Psychiatrist. In J. Corelli (Ed.), *Proceedings of the 3rd World Conference of Therapeutic
Communities* (pp. 263-267). Rome, Centro Italiano di Solidarieta.

Kosten, T.R., Rousaville, B.J. & Kleber, H.D. (1973). Relationship of Depression
to Psychosocial Stressors in Heroin Addicts. *The Journal of Nervous and Mental Disease, 171,* pp. 97-104.

Kraft, A.M. (1962). The Therapeutic Community. In S. Arieti (Ed.), *American Handbook of Psychiatry.*

Kuhn, T. (1962). *The Structure of Scientific Revolution.* Chicago: University of Chicago
Press.

Labouvie, E.W. (1976, December). Longitudinal Designs. In P.M. Bentler, D.J.
Lettieri, & G.A. Austin (Eds.), *Data Analysis Strategies and Designs for Substance Abuse
Research.* Washington, D.C.: U.S. Government Printing Office.

Lakoff, R. (1978). Psychopathology with A Therapeutic Community: A Review of
Psychiatric Consultations from A Drug Addiction Program. *The Addiction Therapist, 2-4,* pp. 48-51.

Langrod, J. & Lowinson, J. (1972). Group Therapy in the Treatment of the Juvenile Narcotic Addict. *International Journal of Pharmacopsychiatry, 7,* pp. 44-52.

LaPorte, D.J., McLellan, A.T., Erdlen, F.R. & Parente, R.J. (1981). Treatment Outcome as A Function of Follow-up difficulty in Substance Abusers. *Journal of Consulting and Clinical Psychology, 49,* pp. 112-119.

Lehman, W.E.K. & Caillouet, S. (1984). Prediction of Behavioral Outcomes 12 Years AFter Treatment. In *Heroin Addiction: 12-Year Posttreatment Follow-up Outcomes.* Symposium conducted at the meeting of the Southwestern Psychological Association, New Orleans.

Lennard, H.L. & Allen, S.D. (1973). The Treatment of Drug Addiction: Toward New Models. *International Journal of Addiction, 8,* pp. 521-535.

Lesser, M.E. (1974). Perceptions of Illness at A Therapeutic Community for Ex-Drug Addicts. "Legitimate Deviancy" or Escape? *Society of Scientific Medicine, 8,* pp. 575-583.

Levy, L.G. (1979). Processes and Activities in Groups. In M. Lieberman & L.D. Borman (Eds.), *Self-Help Groups for Coping with Crisis.* San Francisco: Jossey-Bass.

Lewis, C.E., Rice, J. & Helzer, J.E. (1983). Diagnostic Interactions Alcoholism and Antisocial Personality. *The Journal of Nervous and Mental Disease, 171,* pp. 105-113.

Lewis, S. (1935). *It Can't Happen Here.* Garden City, NY: Doubleday, Doran.

Lieberman, M.A., Yalom, E. & Miles, M.B. (1973). Encounter Groups, First Facts, New York.

Liff, Z.A. (1975). The Charismatic Leader. In Z.A. Liff (Ed.), *The Leader in the Group.* New York: Jason Aronson, p. 119.

Lifton, R. (1979, January 7). The Appeal of the Death Trip. *New York Times Magazine.*

Lindby, K. (1971). Treatment of Drug Addicts in the U.S.A. 1. Synanon, Daytop and Gateway Houses — 3 Therapeutic Communities. *Lakartidningen, 68,* pp. 3505-3516.

Lindesmith, A.R. (1947). *Opiate Addiction.* Bloomington. IN: Indiana University Press.

Lindesmith, A.R. (1965). *The Addict and the Law.* Bloomington, IN: Indiana University Press.

Lindesmith, A.R. (1968). *Addiction and Opiates.* Chicago, IL: Aldine (originally published 1947).

Lipsey, M.W., Cordray, D.S. & Berger D.E. (1981). Evaluation of A Juvenile Diversion Programme: Using Multiple Lines of Evidence. *Evaluation Review, 5,* pp. 282-306.

Locke, J. (1821). *Two Treatises on Government.* London: Printed for R. Butler, W. Reid, W. Sharpe & J. Bumpas, pp. 189-193.

London, P. (1969). *Behavior Control.* New York: Harper & Row, pp. 207-208.

Lowental, U., Wald, D. & Klein, H. (1975). Admission of the Alcoholic into the Therapeutic Community. *Harefuah, 89,* pp. 316-320.

Machiavelli, N. (1940). *The Prince.* In L. Ricci (Trans.) & E.R.P. Vincent (Rev.), New York: Modern Library, Chapter 5.

Maddux, J.F. & Desmond, D. (1975). Rehability and Validity of Information from Heroin Users. *Journal of Psychiatry.* Res. 2, pp. 87-95.

Maertens, J. (1982). Drug-Free Therapeutic Community. *Tijdschr Ziekenverpl, 35,* pp. 221-226.

Main, T.F. (1946). The Hospital as A therapeutic Institution. *Bulletin of the Menninger Clinic, 10.*

Maissie, H.N. (1971). Bedlam in the Therapeutic Community: The Disruption of A Hospital Therapeutic Community as A Pattern of Social Conflict. *Psychiatry-in-Medicine, 2,* pp. 278-293.

Mandel, L., Schulman, J. & Monteriof, R. (1979). A Feminist Approach for One Treatment of Drug-Abusing Women in A Coed Therapeutic Community. *International Journal of Addiction, 14,* pp. 589-597.

Manning, N. (1975). What Happened to the Therapeutic Community. *The Yearbook of Social Policy in Britain.* London: Routledge & Kegan Paul.

Manning, N. (1976). Innovation in Social Policy — The Case of the Therapeutic Community. *Journal of Social Policy, 5,* p. 3.

Manning, N. (1979). The Politics of Survival: The Role of Research in the Therapeutic Community. In Hinshelwood & Manning (Eds.), *Therapeutic Communities.* London: Routledge & Kegan Paul.

Manning, N. & Blake, R. (1979). Implementing Ideals. In Hinshelwood & Manning, (Eds.), *Therapeutic Communities.* London: Routledge & Kegan Paul.

Marlatt, G.A. & Gordon, J.R. (1980). Determinants of Relapse: Implications for the Maintenance of Behavior Change. In P. Davidson & S. Davidson (Eds.), *Behavioral Medicine: Changing Health Lifestyles.* New York: Brunner/Mazel.

McAulliffe, W.E. & Gordon, R.A. (1980). Reinforcement and the Combination of Effects: Summary of A Theory of Opiate Addiction. In D.J. Lettieri, M. Sayers, & H.W. Pearson (Eds.), *Theories on Drug Abuse: Selected Contemporary Perspectives* (NIDA Research Monograph 30). Rockville, MD: NIDA, pp. 137-141.

Menninger, K. (1946). Editor's Comments in Foreword. *Bulletin of the Menninger Clinic, 10*(3).

Meyer-Fehr, P. & Zimmer-Hofler, D. (1983a). Compliance und institutionelle Sozialisation in der Behandlung von delinquenten Heroinabhangigen, Kriminolog. Bull. 1, 1983, S. 29-60.

Meyer-Fehr, P. Zimmer-Hofler, D. (1983b). Soziales und therapeutisches Klima in Therapeutischen Gemeinschaften in: Uchtenhagen, A. und Zimmer-Hofler, D. Eds., 1983 final report to the Swiss National Fund will be edited 1984 by Haupt, Bern.

Miller, R. (1974). Towards A Sociology of Methadone Maintenance. In C. Winick (Ed.), *Sociological Aspects of Drug Dependence.* Cleveland, OH: CRC Press.

Milton, R. & Agrin, A. (1966). Resolution of A Crisis in A Therapeutic Community for Alcoholics. *Quarterly Journal of Studies in Alcohol, 27,* pp. 517-524.

Mitchell, D., Mitchell, C. & Ofshe, R. (1980). *The Light on Synanon: How A Country Weekly Exposed A Corporate Cult — and Won the Pulitzer Prize.* New York: Seaview Books.

Moise, R., Korach, J., Reed, B.G. & Bellows, N. (1982). A Comparison of Black and White Women Entering Drug Abuse Treatment Programmes. *International Journal of Addiction, 17,* pp. 33-49.

Moise, R., Reed, B.G. & Conell, C. (1981). Women in Drug Abuse Treatment Programmes: Factors that Influence Retention at Very Early and Later Stages in Two Treatment Modalities [Summary]. *International Journal of Addiction, 16,* pp. 1295-1300.

Moore, R. & Haugland, S. (1977). Treatment of Alcoholism and Chemical Dependency by Therapeutic Community Approach. *Journal of the Iowa Medical Society, 67,* pp. 477-480.

Moos, R. (1974). *Evaluating Treatment Environments: A Social Ecological Approach.* New York: Wiley.

Moos, R.G. & Finney, J.W. (1983). The Expanding Scope of Alcoholism Treatment Evaluation. *American Psychologist, 38,* pp. 1036-1044.

Moos, R.H. (1974). Underlying Patterns of Treatment Setting in R.H. Moos, *Evaluating Treatment Environments.* New York: Wiley, pp. 326-363.

Morgan, J.N. & Sonquist, J.A. (1963). Problems in the Analysis of Survey Data and A Proposal. *Journal of the American Statistical Association, 58,* pp. 415-35.

Mowrer, O.H. (1977). The Therapeutic Groups and Communities in Retrospect and Prospect. In P. Vamos & J.J. Devlin (Eds.), *Proceedings of the First World Conference on Therapeutic Communities* (pp. 1-62). Montreal, Canada: Portage Press.

Musto, D.F. (1973). *The American Disease: Origins of Narcotic Control.* New Haven, CT: Yale University Press.

Nash, G. (1976). An Analysis of Twelve Studies of the Impact of Drug Abuse Treatment Upon Criminality. In *Drug Use and Crime. Report of the Panel on Drug Use and Criminal Behaviour,* Appendix (NTIS). Washington, D.C.: National Institute on Drug Abuse, pp. 231-271.

Nash, G., Waldorf, D., Foster, J. & Kyllingstadt, A. (1974). The Phoenix House Program. In G. De Leon (Ed.), *Phoenix House: Studies in A Therapeutic Community (1968-73).* New York: MSS Information Corporation.

Nowlis, H. (1975). *Drugs Demystified.* Paris: UNESCO Press.

National Institute on Drug Abuse (1983). *Main Findings for Drug Abuse Treatment Units September 1982* (NIDA Statistical Series, F, No. 10, DHHS Publication No. ADM 83-1284). Rockville, MD: National Institute on Drug Abuse.

Nurco, D. et al. (1975). Studying Addicts Over Time: Methodology and Preliminary Findings. *American Journal of Drug Alcohol Abuse, 2,* pp. 183-196.

O'Brien, W. & Biase, D.V. (1984). The Therapeutic Community: A Current Perspective. *Journal of Psychoactive Drugs, 16*(1), pp. 9-21.

Ogborne, A.C. (1975). The First 100 Residents in A Therapeutic Community for Former Addicts. *British Journal of Addiction, 70,* pp. 65-76.

Ogborne, A.C. (1978). Programme Stability and Resident Turnover in Residential Rehabilitation programmes for alcoholics and Drug Addicts. *British Journal of Addiction, 73,* pp. 47-50.

Ogborne, A.C. & Melotte, C. (1977). An Evaluation of A Therapeutic Community for Former Drug Users. *British Journal of Addiction, 72,* pp. 75-82.

Orlinsky, D.E. & Howard, K.I. (1978). The Relation of Process to Outcome in Psychotherapy. In S.L. Garfield & A.E. Bergin (Eds.) *Handbook of Psychotherapy and Behavior Change: An Empirical Analysis.* New York: John Wiley.

Orne, M.T. (1968). On the Nature of Effective Hope. *International Journal of Psychiatry, 5,* p. 404.

Osgood, C.E., Suci, G.S. & Tannenbaum, P.H. (1957). *The Measurement of Meaning.* Urbana, IL: University of Illinois Press.

Ozbekhan, H. (1975). *Toward A General Theory of Planning Social Systems Sciences Dept.* University of Pennsylvania, The Wharton School.

Pareto, V. (1935). *The Mind and Society.* New York: Harcourt, Brace, p. 2174.

Parsons T. & Smelser, N.J. (1956). *Economy and Society.* Glencoe, IL: Free Press.

Patalano, F. (1976). Psychodiagnostic Testing in A Therapeutic Community for Drug Abusers. *Psychological Reports, 39,* pp. 1279-1285.

Patalano, F. (1978). Personality Dimensions of Drug Abusers Who Enter A Drug-Free Therapeutic Community. *Psychological Reports, 42,* pp. 1063-1069.

Patalano, F. (1980). MMPI Two-Point Code-Type Frequencies of Drug Abusers in A Therapeutic Community. *Psychological Reports, 46,* pp. 1019-1022.

Petzold, H. (1980). Ablosung und Teamarbeit im Four-Steps-Modell der gestalt-therapeutischen Wohngemeinschaften in: Petzold, H. Ed.: Therapeutische Wohngemeinschaften, Pfeiffer, Munchen, 1980.

Pinn, E.J., Martin, J.M. & Walsh, J.F. (1976). A Follow-up Study of 300 Ex-Clients of A Drug-Free Narcotic Treatment Programme in New York City. *American Journal of Drug and Alcohol Abuse, 3,* pp. 397-407.

Platt, J.J., Labate, C. & Wicks, R.J. (1977). *Evaluation Research in Correctional Drug Abuse Treatment.* Lexington: Lexington Books.

Powell, B.J., Penick, E.C., Othmer, E., Bingham, S.F. & Rice, A.S. (1982). Prevalence of Additional Psychiatric Syndromes Among Male Alcoholics. *Journal of Clinical Psychiatry, 43,* pp. 404-407.

Preble, E. & Casey, J.J. Jr. (1969). Taking Care of Business: The Heroin User's Life on the Street. *The International Journal of Addictions, 4*(1), pp. 1-24.

Quinones, M.A., Doyle, K.M., Sheffet, A. & Louria, D.B. (1979). Evaluation of Drug Abuse Rehabilitation Efforts: A Review. *American Journal of Public Health, 69,* pp. 1164-1169.

Rachman, A.W. & Heller, M.E. (1974). Anti-Therapeutic Factors in Therapeutic Communities for Drug Rehabilitation. *Journal of Drug Issues, 4,* pp. 393-403.

Rafaelsen, L. (1974). Alcohol and Drug Abuse Treated in A Therapeutic Community: A Follow-up Study. *Ugesky Laeger, 136,* pp. 1235-1241.

Rawls, J. (1971). *A Theory of Justice.* Cambridge, MA: Harvard University Press.

Relling, Dr. & Roebuck, Dr. (1981, August 29). Therapeutic Communities (Editorial). *The Lancet, 2,* pp. 457-458.

Rinella, V.J. (1976). Proceedings: Rehabilitation or Bust: The Impact of Criminal Justice System Referrals on the Treatment of Drug Addicts and Alcoholics in A Therapeutic Community (Eagleville's Experience). *American Journal of Drug Alcohol Abuse, 3,* pp. 53-58.

Roberts, R.E. (1971). *The New Communes: Coming Together in America.* Englewood Cliffs: Prentice-Hall, Inc.

Rogers, C.R. & Skinner, B.F.(1956). Some Issues Concerning the Control of Human Behavior. *Science, 124,* p. 1057.

Romond, A.M., Forres, C.K. & Kleber, H.D. (1975). Follow-up of Participants in A Drug Dependence Therapeutic Community. *Archives of General Psychiatry, 32,* pp. 369-374.

Rosenthal, M.S. & Biase, D.V. (1969). Phoenix Houses: Therapeutic Communities for Drug Addicts. *Hospital Community Psychiatry, 20,* pp. 26-30.

Rosseau, J.J. (1948). *The Social Contrast.* London: Oxford University Press, pp. 179-180.

Rosser, W.W. (1982). Benzodiazepine Prescription to Middle-Aged Women. *Postgraduate Medicine, 71,* pp. 115-120.

Royer, J.H. (1966). *History of American Socialism.* New York: Dover Publications.

Rubel, J.G., Bratter, T.E., Smirnoff, A.M., Thompson, L.H. & Baker, K.G. (1982). The Role of Structure in the Professional Model and the Self-Help Concept of the Therapeutic Community: Different Strokes for Different Folks? *International Journal of Therapeutic Communities, 3,* pp. 218-230.

Rubin, R.S. (1979). The Community Meeting: A Comparative Study. *American Journal of Psychiatry, 136,* pp. 708-712.

Rucco, J. (1981). The Benevolent Dictator. In G. Leoiselle (Ed.) *6th World Conference of Therapeutic Communities* (pp. 99-100). Manila, Philippines: Astrad Production House.

Rudestam, K.E. & Tarbell, S.E. (1981). The Clinical Judgment Process in the Prescribing of Psychotropic Drugs. *The International Journal of the Addictions, 16,* pp. 1049-1070.

Rutan, J.S. & Rice, C.A. (1981). The Charismatic Leader: Asset or Liability? *Psychotherapy: Theory, Research and Practice, 18* p. 491. Ryan, W. (1971). *Blaming the Victim.* New York: Pantheon.

Saari, C. (1976). *Affective Symbolization in the Dynamics of Character Disordered Functioning, 46*(2). Smith College Studies in Social Work, pp. 70-113.

Sacks, J.G. & Levy, N.M. (1979). Objective Personality Changes in Residents of A Therapeutic Community. *American Journal of Psychiatry, 136,* pp. 796-799.

Sansome, J. (1980). Retention Patterns in A Therapeutic Community for the Treatment of Drug Abuse. *International Journal of Addiction, 15* pp. 711-736.

Santayana, G. (1920). *Character and Opinion in the United States.* London: Constable, p. 87.

Sarns, H.W. (1958). *Autobiography of Brook Farm.* Englewood Cliffs, NJ: Prentice-Hall.

Scanlon, J.C. (1976). Proceedings: Cost Savings/Benefit Analysis of Drug Abuse Treatment. *American Journal of Drug Alcohol Abuse, 3,* pp. 95-101.

Schacter, S. (1952). Comment. *American Journal of Sociology, 57,* pp. 554-62.

Schur, E.M. (1973). *Radical Nonintervention.* Englewood Cliffs, NJ: Prentice-Hall.

Schweitzer, A. (1950). *The Philosophy of Civilization.* New York: Macmillan., pp. 154-155.

SNF (1977). Schweizerischer Nationalfonds zur Forderung der wissenschaftlichen Forschung. Jahresbericht 1977, 32-38 und 132-136.

Seashore, S.E. (1954). *Group Cohesiveness in the Industrial Work Group.* Ann Arbor, MI: Survey Research Center.

Sechrest, L. & Redner, R. (1979). *How Well Does It Work? Review of Criminal Justice Evaluation, 1978.* Washington, D.C.: Institute of Law Enforcement and Criminal Justice.

Sells, S.B. (1974). *The Effectiveness of Drug Abuse Treatment, 1-2.* Cambridge, MA: Ballinger Publishing Co.

Sells, S.B. (1977, October). *Evaluation of Treatment for Drug Dependence. Overview and Rationale for Outcome Evaluation.* Paper presented at the Seventh International Institute on the Prevention and Treatment of Drug Dependence. Lisbon, Portugal.

Sells, S.B. (1979). Treatment Effectiveness. In R.I. DuPont, A. Goldstein and J. O'Donnell, (Eds.), *Handbook on Drug Abuse.* Washington, D.C.: National Institute on Drug Abuse, pp. 105-118.

Sells, S.B. & Simpson, D.D. (Eds.) (1976). *The Effectiveness of Drug Abuse Treatment, 3-5.* Cambridge, MA: Ballinger.

Sells, S.B. Simpson, D. & Joe, G. (1976). A National Follow-up Study to Evaluate The Effectiveness of Drug Abuse Treatment. *American Journal of Drug Alcohol Abuse, 3,* pp. 545-556.

Sells, S.B., Simpson, D.D. Joe, G., Demaree, R., Savage, L. & Lloyd, M.A. (1976). A National Follow-up Study to Evaluate the Effectiveness of Drug Abuse Treatment. A Report of Cohort 1 of the DARP 5 Years Later. *American Journal of Drug Alcohol Abuse, 3,* pp. 545-556.

Selvin, H.C. & Hagstrom, W.O. (1963). The Empirical Classification of Formal Groups. *American Sociological Review, 28,* pp. 399-411.

Shapiro, M.H. (1972). The Uses of Behavior Control Technologies: A Response. *Issues in Cirminology, 7,* p. 55.

Sharaf, M.R. (1974). Phoenix House: Psychopathological Signs among Male & Female Drug-Free Residents. *Addictive Disorders, 1,* pp. 135-151.

Shelley, J.A. & Bassin, A. (1964). Daytop Lodge: Halfway House for Drug Addicts. *Federal Probation, 28,* pp. 46-54.

Shelley, J.A. & Bassin, A. (1965). Daytop Lodge: A New Treatment Approach for Drug Addicts. *Corrective Psychiatry, 11,* pp. 186-195.

Siegler, M. & Osmond, H. (1968). Models of Drug Addiction. *International Journal of the Addiction, 3,* pp. 3-24.

Simpson, D.D. (1979). The Relation of Time Spent in Drug Abuse Treatment to Posttreatment Outcomes. American Journal of Psychiatry, 136, pp. 1449-1453.

Simpson, D.D. (1981). Treatment for Drug Abuse: Follow-up Outcomes and Length of Time Spent. *Archives of General Psychiatry, 38*(8), pp. 875-880.

Simpson, D.D. (1984). National Treatment System Evaluation Based on the DARP Follow-up Research. In F. Tims & J. Ludford (Eds.) *Drug Abuse Treatment Evaluation: Strategies, Progress, and Prospects* (NIDA Research Analysis and Utilization System (RAUS) Monograph Series). Washington, D.C.: U.S. Government Printing Office.

Simpson, D.D. & Joe, G.W. (1977). *Sample Design and Data Collection: National Follow-up Study of Admissions to Drug Abuse Treatment in the DARP During 1969-1972.* (IBR Report 77-8). College Station: Behavioral Research Program, Texas A&M University.

Simpson,D.D., Joe, G.W., Lehman, W.E.K. & Sells, S.B. (1985). Addiction Careers: Etiology, Treatment, and 12-Year Follow-up Outcomes. *Journal of Drug Issues.*

Simpson, D.C., Lloyd, M.R. & Gent, N.N.J. (1977). *Reliability and Validity of Data* (Institute of Behavioural Research, Report 76-81). Fort Worth, TX: Christian University, Institute of Behavioural Research.

Simpson, D.D. & Savage, L.J. (1980). Drug Abuse Treatment Readmission and Outcomes: Three Year Follow-up of DARP Patients. *Archives of General Psychiatry, 37*(8), pp. 896-901.

Simpson, D.D., Savage, L.J., Lloyd, M.R. & Sells, S.B. (1977). *Evaluation of Drug Abuse Treatments Based on the First Year After DARP* (Institute of Behavioral Research, Report 77-14). Fort Worth, TX: Texas Christian University, Institute of Behavioural Research.

Simpson, D.D. & Sells, S.B. (1982). Effectiveness of Treatment for Drug Abuse: An Overview of the DARP Research Program. *Advances in Alcohol and Substance Abuse, 2*(1), pp. 7-29.

Siroka, R.W., Siroka, E.K. & Schloss, G.A. (1971). *Sensitivity Training and Group Encounter.* New York: Grosseth and Dunlop, Inc.

Sirotnik, K.A. & Bailey, R.C (1975). A Cost-Benefit Analysis of A Multimodality Heroin Treatment Project. *International Journal of Addiction, 10,* pp. 443-451.

Sk'ala, J., Matov'a, A., Hrodkov'a, J. & Homolkov'a, J. (1973). Marking System and Therapeutic Community. *Cesk Psychiatr, 69,* pp. 303-309.

Skinner, H.A. (1981). Assessment of Alcohol Problems: Basic Principles, Critical Issues and Future Trends. In Y. Israel et al. (Eds.), *Research Advances in Alcohol and Drug Problems, 6.* New York: Plenum Press.

Skolnick, N.J. & Zuckerman, M. (1979). Personality Change in Drug Abusers: A Comparison of Therapeutic Community and Prison Groups. *Journal of Consulting and Clinical Psychology, 47,* pp. 768-770.

Slotkin, E.J. & Senay, E.C. (1973). *Gateway's Success in the Rehabilitation of Drug Abusers.* Chicago: Gateway Houses.

Smart, R.G. (1976). Outcome Studies of Therapeutic Community and Halfway House Treatment for Addicts. *International Journal of Addiction, 11,* pp. 143-159.

Sobel, B.S. (1976). Combined Tertiary Prevention: The Existence and Treatment Together of the Addiction/Mental Health Interface. In D.J. Ottenberg & E.L. Carpey (Eds.) *Proceedings of the 8th Annual Eagleville Conference on Alcoholism and Drug Addiction: Critical Issues in Hard Times.* New York: Marcel Dekker, pp. 145-154. (Special issue of the American Journal of Drug and Alcohol Abuse, 3(1), 1976).

Sobel, B.S. (1979). *Psychopharmacologic Medications as Used in Treatment with the Addictive Person.* Unpublished Manuscript. (Available from Bernard S. Sobel, D.O., Director of Psychiatry, Valley Forge Medical Center, 1033 W. Germantown Pike, Norristown, Pennsylvania, 19403).

Sobel, B.S. (1981, September). *Substance Use Disorders with (Other) Psychiatric Illness: Interface, Issues, and Problems.* Paper presented at the International Congress on Drugs and Alcohol, Jerusalem, Israel.

Sobel, B.S. & Antes, D. (1975, November). *The Borderline Alcoholic Addict: Assessment, Criteria, Treatment in the Abstinence Therapeutic Community.* Paper presented at the Americana College of Neuropsychiatry, Las Vegas, NV.

Sonquist, J.A. & Morgan, J.N. (1964). *The Detection of Interaction Effects* (Monograph No. 35). University of Michigan, Survey Research Center, Institute for Social Research.

Stanton, M.D. & Todd, T.T. (1982). *The Family Therapy of Drug Abuse and Addiction.* London: Guilford Press.

Stephens, R.C. & McBridge, D.C. (1976, Spring). Becoming A Street Addict. *Human Organizations, 35*(1), pp. 87-93.

Stine, L.J., Patrick, S.W. & Molina, J. (1982). What is the Role of Violence in the Therapeutic Community? *International Journal of Addiction, 17*, pp. 377-392.

Stotland, E. (1969). *The Psychology of Hope: An Integration of Experimental, Clinical, and Social Approaches*. San Francisco: Jossey-Bass, Inc.

Street, D. (1965). The Inmate Group in Custodial and Treatment Settings. *American Sociological Review, 30*, pp. 40-45.

Sugarman, B. (1974). *Daytop Village: A Therapeutic Community*. New York: Holt, Rinehart and Winston, pp. 129-130.

Sugarman, B. (in press). Towards A New, Common Model of the Therapeutic Community: Structural Components, Learning Processes and Outcomes. *International Journal of Therapeutic Communities* in press.

Susman, R.M. (1975). Drug Abuse, Congress and the Fact-Finding Process. *Annals, 417*, pp. 16-26.

Sutker, P.B., Allain, A.N., Smith, C.J. & Cohen, G.H. (1978). Addict Descriptions of Therapeutic Community, Multimodality and Methadone Maintenance Treatment Clients and Staff. *Journal of Consulting and Clinical Psychology, 46*, pp. 508-517.

Tarry, C. & Wilk, R. (1970, September 11). Addicts in A Therapeutic Community. *Nursing Mirror, 131*, pp. 32-34.

Thoreau, H.D. (1899). *Walden or, Life in the Woods*. Boston: Houghton Mifflin.

Tims, F. & Ludford, J. (Eds.) (1984). *Drug Abuse Treatment Evaluation: Strategies, Progress, and Prospects* (NIDA) Research Analysis and Utilization System (RAUS) Monograph Series). Washington, D.C.: U.S. Government Printing Office.

Tittle, C.R. & Hill, R.J. (1967). Attitude Measurement and Prediction of Behavior: An Evaluation of Conditions and Measurement Techniques. *Sociometry, 30*, pp. 199-213.

Tolbert, C. (1980). Fiscal Crisis in A Therapeutic Community. *International Journal of Addiction, 15*, pp. 1011-1019.

Tonnies, F. (1957). *Community and Society (Gemenischaft and Gellschaft)*. East Lansing, Michigan State University Press (translated by C.P. Loomis).

Torrey, E.F. (1974). *The Death of Psychiatry*. Radnor, PA: Chilton Book Company.

Treffert, D.A. & Sack, M. (1973). A Drug Unit for Life-Style Change: The Tellurian Community. *Hospital Community Psychiatry, 24*, pp. 36-40.

Trist, E.L. (1973). Collaborative Social and Technical Innovation. In F.E. Emery & E.L. Trist (Eds.), *Towards A Social Ecology*. London: Plenum Press.

Trist, E.L., Higgins, G.W., Murray, H. & Pollack, A.B. (1963). *Organizational Choice*. London: Tavistock.

Uchtenhagen, A. & Zimmer-Hofler, D. (1981). Theoretisches Model zur Unterpretation Devianter Karrieren, in: Papers presented at the 11th International Institute on the Prevention & Treatment of Drug Dependence, Vienna, Ed. E. Tongue, ICAA Publ., Lausanne.

Uchtenhagen, A. & Zimmer-Hofler, D. (1983). Final report to the Swiss National Fund on Scientific Research will be edited in 1984 by Haupt, Bern.

Vaglumn, P. (1981). What Was Helpful and What Was Harmful? Patients Evaluate the Progress of Recovery in A Therapeutic Community. *Journal of Oslo City Hospital, 31*, pp. 55-58.

Vaglum, P. & Bjelke, B. (1973, January 10). Young Drug Addicts in A Psychiatric Department. Body Conditions and Reactions on Meeting A Therapeutic Community. *Tidsskr Nor Laegenforen, 93,* pp. 7-12.

Vaillant, G. (1966). Twelve Year Follow-up of New York Narcotic Addicts. American Journal of Psychiatry, 123, pp. 573-584.

Vaillant, G.E. (1966). A 12-Year Follow-up of New York Narcotic Addicts: The Relation of Treatment to Outcome. *American Journal of Psychiatry, 122,* pp. 727-737.

Vaillant, G. (1973). A 20-Year Follow-up of New York Narcotic Addicts. *Archives of General Psychiatry, 29,* pp. 237-241.

VanStone, W.W. & Gilbert, R. (1972). Peer Confrontation Groups: What, Why and Whether. *American Journal of Psychiatry, 129,* pp. 583-589.

Veysey, L. (1973). *The Commune Experience: Anarchist and Mystical Counter-Cultures in America.* New York: Harper & Row, p. 15.

Volkman, R. & Cressey, D.R. (1963). Differential Association and the Rehabilitation of Drug Addicts. *American Journal of Sociology, 69,* pp. 129-42.

Volkman, R. & Cressey, D. (1966). Differential Associations and the Rehabilitation of Drug Addicts. In J. O'Donnell & J.C. Ball, (Eds.), *Narcotic Addiction.* New York: Harper and Row, pp. 209-233.

Vos, H. (1983, May). *Separational Conflicts and Their Impact on the Therapeutic Community,* paper presented at the 7th World Conference of Therapeutic Communities, Chicago.

Waldorf, D. (1971). Social Control in Therapeutic Communities for the Treatment of Drug Addicts. *International Journal of Addiction, 6,* pp. 29-43.

Waldorf, D (1973). *Careers in Dope.* Englewood Cliffs, NJ: Prentice-Hall.

Washburne, N. (1977). *Dynamics of Treatment in Therapeutic Communities* (Technical Report No 5). Rutgers University.

Webb, R.A. & Bruen, W.J. (1967-1968). Multiple Child-Parent Therapy in A Family Therapeutic Community. *International Journal of Social Psychiatry, 14,* pp. 50-55.

Weber, M. (1947). *The Theory of Social and Economic Organization.* Oxford: Oxford University Press, pp. 328-329. (translated by A.M. Henderson & T. Parsons)

Weppner, R.S. (1973). Some Characteristics of an Ex-Addict Self-Help Therapeutic Community and its Members. *British Journal of Addiction, 68,* pp. 73-79, 243-250.

Weppner, R.S. (1976). The Complete Participant: Problems in Participants Observation in A Therapeutic Community. *Addictive Disorders, 2,* pp. 643-658.

Weppner, R.S. (1983). *The Untherapeutic Community: Organizational Behavior in a Failed Addiction Treatment Program.* Lincoln, NB: University of Nebraska Press, p. 227.

Wexler, H.K. & De Leon, G. (1977). The Therapeutic Community: Mutli-variate Prediction of Retention. *American Journal of Drug Alcohol Abuse, 4,* p. 2.

Wheeler, S. (1961). Socialization in Correctional Communities. *American Sociological Review, 26,* pp. 699-712.

Whiteley, J. (1979). Progress and Reflection. In Hinshelwood & Manning (Eds.), *Therapeutic Communities.* London: Routledge & Kegan Paul.

Wilson, A.T.M., Trist, E.L. & Curle, A. (1952). Transitional Communities and Social Re-Connection: A Study of Civil Resettlement of British Prisoners of War. In G.E. Swanson, et al. (Ed.), *Readings in Social Psychology.* New York: Holt.

Wilson, S. (1978). The Effect of Treatment in A Therapeutic Community on Intravenous Drug Abuse. *British Journal of Addiction, 73*, pp. 407-411.

Wilson, S. & Mandelbrote B. (1978). The Relationship Between Duration of Treatment in A Therapeutic Community for Abusers and Subsequent Criminality. *British Journal of Psychology, 132*, pp. 487-491.

Winick, C. (1962). Maturing Out of Narcotic Addiction. *Bulletin On Narcotics, 14*, pp. 107.

Winick, C. (1974). *Sociological Aspects of Drug Dependence.* Cleveland, OH: CRC Press.

Winick, C. (1980). An Empirical Asessment of Therapeutic Communities in New York City. In L. Brill & C. Winick (Eds.), *Yearbook of Substance Use and Abuse.* New York: Human Sciences Press.

Wolberg, A.R. (1975). The Leader and Society. In Z.A. Liff (Ed.), *The Leader in the Group.* New York: Jason Aronson, pp. 249-250.

Wolf, A. & Schwartz, E.K. (1975). The Leader and the Homogeneous or Heterogeneous Group. In Z.A. Liff, (Ed.), *The Leader in the Group.* New York: Jason Aronson, p. 47.

Wolfe, T. (1936). *The Story of A Novel.* New York: Charles Scribner's, p. 39.

Woody, G.E., O'Brien, C.P. & Greenstein, R. (1978). Multimodality Treatment of Narcotic Addiction: An Overview. National Institute of Drug Abuse Research Monograph Series, 19, pp. 226-240.

Yablonsky, L. (1963). The Anticriminal Society: Synanon. *Federal Probation, 26*, pp. 50-57.

Yablonsky, L. (1965). *Synanon: The Tunnel Back.* New York: Macmillan.

Yablonsky, L. (1970). *Synanon: The Tunnel Back.* New York: Macmillan.

Yalom, I. (1975). *The Theory and Practice of Group Psychotherapy.* New York: Basic Books.

Zarcone, V.P., Jr. (1980). An Eclectic Therapeutic Community for the Treatment of Addiction. *International Journal of Addiction, 15*,pp. 515-528.

Ziegenfuss, J.T. (1977, October). The Therapeutic Community as A Model for Implementing Patient's Rights. *Journal of Clinical Psychology, 33*, p. 4.

Zeigenfuss, J.T. (1980). The Therapeutic Community: A Plan for Continued International Development. *International Journal of Therapeutic Communities, 1*(2).

Ziegenfuss, J.T. & Gaughan-Fickes, J. (1976, August). Alternative to Prison Programs and Client Civil Rights: A Question. *Contemporary Drug Problems.*

Zimber, S. (1978). Treatment of the Elderly Alcoholic in the Community and in an Institutional Setting. *Addictive Disorders, 3*, pp. 417-427.

Zimmer-Hofler, D. (1981a). Interviewing Heroin Addicts for Research. In W.R. Minsel & W. Herff, Methodology in Psychotherapy Research *Proceedings of the 1st European Conference on Psychotherapy Research* (pp. 60-69). Frankfurt: Peter Lang.

Zimmer-Hofler, D. & Widmer, A. (1981). *Democratically or Hierarchically Structured Therapeutic Community for Heroin Addicts?* Paper presented at the 6th World Conference of Therapeutic Communities, Manila.

Zimmer-Hofler, D., Meyer-Fehr, P. & Widmer, A. (1982). Opiatabhangige in therapeutischen Gemeinschaften. *Drogenreport, 3*, pp. 1-23.

Zimmer-Hofler, D. & Meyer-Fehr, P. (1983). What Can Researchers Learn From A

Therapeutic Community? What Can A Therapeutic Community Learn From Research? Vortragsmanuskript, Chicago.

Zuckerman, M., Sola, S., Masterson, J. & Angelone, J.V. (1975). MMPI Patterns in Drug Abusers Before and After Treatment in Therapeutic Communities. *Journal of Consulting and Clinical Psychology, 43,* pp. 286-296.